This document is geared towards providing exact and reliable information in regards to the topic and issue covered. The publication is sold with the idea that the publisher is not required to render accounting, officially permitted, or otherwise, qualified services. If advice is necessary, legal or professional, a practiced individual in the profession should be ordered.

From a Declaration of Principles which was accepted and approved equally by a Committee of the American Bar Association and a Committee of Publishers and Associations.

The information provided herein is stated to be truthful and consistent, in that any liability, in terms of inattention or otherwise, by any usage or abuse of any policies, processes, or directions contained within is the solitary and utter responsibility of the recipient reader. Under no circumstances will any legal responsibility or blame be held against the publisher for any reparation, damages, or monetary loss due to the information herein, either directly or indirectly.

Respective authors own all copyrights not held by the publisher.

The trademarks that are used are without any consent, and the publication of the trademark is without permission or backing by the trademark owner. All trademarks and brands within this book are for clarifying purposes only and are the owned by the owners themselves, not affiliated with this document.

Table of Contents

Introduction

I had a problem following the keto diet when I first started. Personally, it is not easy for a big guy like me to suddenly ditch carbs and start this diet. I am a steak kind of guy but not without my mashed potatoes. I also enjoy eating sweet desserts after every meal, so I didn't see it as possible for me to follow this particular diet.

Now that you know about the science behind how the ketogenic diet works, it is time that you learn the art of maintaining the diet. If you are thinking that all there is to it is to eat more lean proteins and fatty food to push your body into ketosis, you would be missing out, there is so much more to this diet than just chowing down an entire roasted pig day in and day out.

While I was convinced by the science part of the ketogenic diet, somehow, I was apprehensive about following the diet. How would I be able to sustain this particular diet if I restrict myself from eating carbs? Would it change the way I do grocery shopping or prepared my meals? These are some of the questions that I asked myself before starting this diet.

I understand that some of you reading about the ketogenic diet may have doubts on how to go about this diet. But it is easy as long as you have the right guide, and plan your meals. Planning is the key to success and happiness. I believe this is also true when you plan your diet and weight loss journey.

While you might think that you have to exert extra effort to plan your ketogenic meals, all your hard work will eventually pay off. It might take some time getting used to, but if you develop the habit and discipline, following the ketogenic diet can be as natural as breathing.

I had to discover everything about the ketogenic diet on my own. I want to share my success with you so that you can also lose weight effectively. Thus, let this book serve as your guide in what you need to know about ketogenic diet meal preparation and be amazed by its simplicity.

The Basic of Meal Prep

Meal prepping is simply preparing your meals ahead of time. It is like having your own TV dinner when and where you want it. The only difference is that you know what goes into your food and you ensure that all ingredients are compliant with the principles of the ketogenic diet.

While it might sound like you have to exert a little extra effort in making your meals, it will greatly help you succeed. I can guarantee that meal prepping will save you time, money, and energy. Moreover, it will also increase your chances of sticking to the diet.

The Benefits of Meal Prepping

Planning is king when it comes to sticking to any diet. Research shows that planning–in all aspects–can increase your chances of following through on what you need to do. In a study published in the *British Journal of Health Psychology,* those who schedule their workout pushed through with their plans successfully. The same is true when following the ketogenic diet. If you are still not convinced, these benefits will surely win you over on doing meal prep.

- **Helps to avoid decision fatigue:** Decision fatigue happens when you get tired of making decisions about anything – in this case, the type of food that you will eat every day. Did you know that making decisions daily about what food to it can reduce your willpower? The reason why many people get tired of the ketogenic diet easily is that they have to decide every day what to eat and what to avoid. So, if you plan your meals ahead of time, you reduce your choices, so you don't need to go through planning daily because you have already decided ahead of time what you are going to eat on any particular day. This frees up a lot of mental space so that you can focus on other things that need your attention.

- **Saves you time and energy:** Many people make an excuse that they cannot follow through with the ketogenic diet because they don't have enough time and energy to prepare their meals. But meal prep can solve this problem as you only have to commit a few hours each week to prepare everything from planning, shopping, and cooking meals.

- **Grocery shopping is easier:** Since planning ahead allows you to know what ingredients you will use to make your meals; grocery shopping becomes a breeze. All you need to do is to make a list and you are good to go.

- **Saves you money:** Meal prepping can also save you a lot of money. It is so easy to waste food if you don't have a plan. With meal prep, you can plan what you can make with all the ingredients you have. It ensures that everything that you buy will be used, thus saving money in the process.

- **Helps to achieve ketosis successfully:** Perhaps one of the most difficult things when following the ketogenic diet is to stick with ketosis. Since you are still eating something while following this diet, it is important that you keep track of your micros to ensure that you are not eating beyond the recommended amount of carbs or not eating too much protein. This is the reason why calculating your macros is really important. While doing this can be painstaking if you eat food randomly, this can be achieved easily if you plan ahead. Since everything has already been calculated for you, it makes things much easier and you don't have to keep track of your macros every time you eat.

Tips and Tricks for Keto Meal Prep

Successful keto meal prepping requires planning and preparation. When I started out, I discovered things along the way. I don't want you to experience the same things I did. Thus, below are helpful tips and tricks that you can follow when doing keto meal prepping.

- **Determine your goal:** You want to lose weight. That's why you decided to take on this particular diet. But what is exactly your goal? Be specific. Do you want to 20 pounds in 4 months? Do you want to develop healthy, clean eating habits? Do you want to follow a plant-based ketogenic diet (hey, it is possible!)? By determining your goal, you will be able to design a meal plan that works for you.

- **Use a spreadsheet:** If you want to be successful while following this diet regimen, make sure that you plan ahead. What better way to do it than to embrace your inner nerd—by using a spreadsheet. Use a spreadsheet not only to plan your meals but also to calculate your macros and create your weekly grocery list. There are so many things that you can do with a spreadsheet to organize not only your groceries but also yourself. Take a screenshot of your spreadsheet and take it with you when you are ready to do your grocery shopping.

- **Go easy when planning your meals:** While you have the luxury to plan and make very sophisticated meals so that your palate will not be bored, I recommend that you go easy when it comes to choosing your meals. If it is your first time to do keto meal prepping, you might want to choose simple recipes so that you will not be overwhelmed with the meal prepping itself.

- **Choose a day for meal prepping:** Dedicate a specific day when you will do all the necessary meal preparations for your week. I usually do meal prepping on the weekends because that is when I have more free time. But any day that works for you is fine.

- **Stock your kitchen with the right equipment:** You might think that meal prepping is easy but if you don't have the right equipment, things can be difficult. You don't need special knives or bulky kitchen appliances. What you need the most for meal prepping are reusable containers. Stock up on as many containers as you can to store your food. Lastly, make sure that you have a lot of space in your fridge to store your food.

- **Know your macros:** When choosing the recipes that you want to prepare, make sure that you know your macros. If you don't know how to calculate your macros, there are macro calculators online that you can use. I use this <u>Macronutrient Calculator</u>.

- **Use a slow cooker or a Dutch oven:** If you are cooking bag batches of food particularly protein, it may be wise to use a Dutch oven or a slow cooker so that you save energy when cooking as you leave the food to cook on its own—no stirring needed.

- **Skipping breakfast might be a good idea:** Although this is not directly related to meal prepping, skipping breakfast means that you will have one less meal to pack. Moreover, skipping breakfast pushes the body into ketosis so you get benefits just as you would with the ketogenic diet.

Common Keto Meal Prep Mistakes You Must Know

Preparing meals ahead of time can help you achieve your weight loss goals. But even if you have already mastered the art of meal prepping, you are still prone to making mistakes. Mistakes in meal prepping are not only costly and a waste of effort but this should not discourage you. Avoid these common meal prepping mistakes so that you will enjoy your keto-compliant meals.

- **Discounting your macros:** Remember that the ketogenic diet is based on the consumption of healthy fats to drive ketosis. But if you are leaning towards one macro–particularly protein–it stops your body from undergoing ketosis. As a general rule, you need 60-75% of calories from fat, 15-30% of calories from protein and a very minimal amount of carbs. Remember that and you are good to go.

- **Making all your meals in one day:** The problem with doing meal prepping in one day is that you will have to store your meals in the fridge for several days. What if you need to prepare a large batch enough for seven days? Remember that food goes bad after three or five days even if they are stored in the fridge. Thus, prepping a couple of times throughout the week can ensure that your meals taste fresher compared to when you prepare them once a week. But if you don't have the luxury of time and you can only prepare once every week, you can freeze some meals to reduce the risk of spoilage and to make them last longer.

- **Not mixing things up:** Eating the same meals every day can be boring. For instance, if you prepared roasted chicken good for 4 days, you might lose your appetite when you eat roasted chicken day in and day out. Part of planning for meal prep is to prepare other food items so you can mix and match. This helps keep diet boredom at bay.

- **Your kitchen is not well-equipped:** Meal prepping can be overwhelming because you have to prepare larger batches of food than you would normally cook. If your kitchen is not equipped for making large batches of food, it could be difficult for you to meal prep. Your kitchen should be equipped with options for pots, pans, and containers but also your kitchen should have your go-to staple ingredients on hand. Stock up on spices, condiments, oils, and other ingredients that are necessary to make ketogenic-friendly meals.

- **Not choosing simple recipes:** You can save a lot of time if you choose recipes with just a few ingredients as well as recipes that require similar ingredients. It makes a shorter shopping list and speeds up cooking time, so that you don't get overwhelmed with all the chopping and cooking.

- **Making things complicated:** Meal prepping should never be complicated. One of the biggest mistakes that people make is fussing over cooking and employing complicated cooking techniques. If you are a kitchen newb like me, I recommend that you use a crockpot. You can literally dump all your ingredients into the pot and forget about it, while they cook.

- **Not storing food properly:** The containers that you use when storing your meals can affect your food. Make sure that your containers are adequate in size to help keep your portions under control. Aside from the size of the containers, it is also important to choose containers that are airtight. Otherwise the food can become soggy or go stale easily. If you commute to work, you can store your food in a mini cooler so that it doesn't spoil before its time to eat your lunch.

How to Meal Prep Like A Pro

Meal prepping should not be overwhelming. There is a way to prepare meals like a pro. Believe me, I learned several valuable lessons in meal prep when I was starting out with this diet. Let me stress to you, that preparing meals in advance like a pro does not come with standard steps. Everyone meal preps their food differently. Below are some basic steps to get you started, feel free to follow them when making keto-friendly meals.

#1 – Decide What You Want to Eat

The most important step in meal prepping is deciding which foods you want to eat for the upcoming week. Allocate one day of your week to sit down and create a meal outline. This will help you plan what you want to eat in the next few days. Deciding on which foods to prepare can be tough. There are so many recipes out there that you can try. Let me help you decide based on the questions below:

- **What meals do you want to eat every day of the week?** Create a weekly table for breakfast, lunch, dinner, and snacks and write down foods or recipes that you want to eat each day.
- **How many people will be eating the meals?** If you are making recipes for the entire family, you may need to adjust the amount of food that you are making to accommodate all family members.
- **Is the recipe simple?** If you are a kitchen novice, there is no point in making meals that are difficult.

#2 – Shop for Ingredients

Once you have created a meal plan and decided on which recipes to make, the next thing that you need to do is to write down all ingredients that the recipe requires. Organizing your grocery list will make it easier for you to shop for the things that you need. Once you have a grocery list, decide on which days you will shop for the ingredients. You can either break up your shopping excursion or complete it in one day. It is up to you.

When shopping, break your trip down by food categories so that it is easier to find the ingredients that you need. For instance, if you are shopping for red meat, buy chicken if it is included in your list. Follow your list and stick to it.

#3 – Cook Your Meals

Once you have all the ingredients that you need, it is time to cook your meals. Cooking your meals can be tricky especially if you are still starting out but it will get better with practice. Take note that there is no standard rule to follow when meal prepping but there are things that you can do to make cooking easier.

Read the recipes and identify which ones take the longest time to make. Start with those recipes so that you can multitask and do the other simpler recipes. For instance, if you are cooking slow cooked chicken, you can cook the chicken first then make the cauliflower rice while the chicken is inside the crockpot.

Do all your preparations before starting to cook. This means chop and measure all ingredients for each recipe so that you don't waste a lot of time. Getting organized in the kitchen is key in meal prepping.

Once the meals are cooked, place them in separate containers so that they are ready to go. Make sure that you label each container with the name of the meal and the date when you made it, so that you know which ones to consume first.

While some people recommend that you mix and match different recipes so that you can just grab them from the fridge and eat, I don't necessarily advise it because the flavors will be all over the place and it might make the food less appetizing. What I do suggest is that once you are ready to eat, take a serving from each container and place in one container before heating everything up.

Meal Prep Principles for A Healthy Keto Lifestyle

The ketogenic diet is one of the best diets to support a healthy weight. But this does not mean that you can get away with eating any foods rich in fat and protein. If you want to live a healthy keto lifestyle, it is important that you apply the basic principles of meal prepping so that achieving the right results is easy.

Sourcing Ingredients

The most important principle with keto meal prepping is sourcing your ingredients. Just because the ketogenic diet is laden with fat does not mean that you can use any ingredients. You will get more benefit if you source whole food ingredients.

Source out high-quality fats, grass-fed meats, and wild seafood. Opt for foods that are not made in a processing plant. They come with a lot of additives particularly sugar and/or salt. For ingredients that will increase your fat intake such as coconut oil, MCT oil, olive oil, lard, and ghee, always keep a stock in your pantry and buy them especially when they happen to be on sale.

Always Use A Meal Template

Using a meal plan template of the recipes that you are planning to cook will ensure your success in following the ketogenic diet. Create several columns in the template and write a shopping list in one section while the recipe goes to another column. The other sections you can use to put in other important notes such as the macros, equipment needed, and schedule so that your meal template will have all the information that you need to successfully do meal prepping.

Shopping Trips

Another challenging part of the keto meal prep is shopping for the ingredients. Plan trips that will work with your schedule. Remember that your life does not revolve around dieting and meal prepping, so you need to work around your schedule. If you work full time, shop over the weekend. Avoid the rush hour by doing your shopping early.

Meal Prep FAQs

I took the liberty of compiling some possible FAQs about meal prepping.

1.) Do I need to freeze everything?

Unless you are making large batches of food that need to last until the end of the week and you want them to last longer, you may store the ready-made meals in the fridge.

2.) How long before the food gets bad?

Food often lasts between 3 and 5 days when stored in the fridge. However, it can stay longer inside the freezer. Knowing this, you can prep fewer meals than needed or divide your meal prepping into twice a week.

3.) How long does it take to meal prep?

There is no definite time on how long meal prepping lasts. It varies depending on the types of food that you make or if you have help in the kitchen.

4.) How much food should I prepare?

The amount of food that you prepare largely depends on your caloric needs as well as if other family members are also following the ketogenic diet. Make sure that you make the necessary adjustments when following a recipe.

5.) Will it get boring to eat the same food every day?

The answer is no especially if you know how to mix and match your food. I recommend that you prepare different dishes so that you can mix different types of food every meal.

Keto Meal-Prep Breakfast Recipes
Beef and Egg White Scramble

Servings per Recipe: 4
Cooking Time: 20 minutes

Ingredients:
- Salt and pepper to taste
- ½ cup red peppers, chopped
- 4 small tomatoes, chopped
- 2 cups baby spinach
- 8 egg whites
- 1-lb lean ground beef
- Cooking spray

Directions:
1. Heat a non-stick pan over medium heat.
2. Sprat with cooking spray and add beef to the hot skillet.
3. Stir constantly to break the larger pieces. Let it cook for 10 minutes until no longer pink and juices have dried.
4. In a separate bowl, beat the egg whites until fluffy. Add salt and pepper to taste.
5. Pour over the beef and add the vegetables on top of beef and egg mixture. Cover.
6. Continue cooking on low fire for 10 minutes until the eggs are set.
7. Evenly divide into suggested servings, let it cool, and store in meal prep ready container.

Nutrition Information:
Calories per serving: 310; Protein: 38.7g; Fat: 14.1g; Carbohydrates: 5.3g; Fiber: 1.7g

Breakfast Muffin Cups

Servings per Recipe: 3
Cooking Time: 15 minutes

Ingredients:
- Salt and pepper to taste
- 2 tbsp red onion, finely chopped
- Sprig of fresh basil
- 1 cup shredded Mozzarella cheese
- 3 tbsp red pepper
- ½ cup sliced spinach
- 6 slices shaved turkey ham
- 6 large eggs
- Cooking spray or olive oil

Directions:
1. Spray a non-stick muffin pan with olive oil.
2. In each muffin cup, drape a piece of a turkey ham to make a cup.
3. Crack an egg and pour it gently in the turkey cup.
4. Add a little bit of vegetables on top of the egg.
5. Garnish with shredded mozzarella cheese and chopped basil. Add salt and pepper to taste.
6. Put the muffin tin in the oven that is preheated to 350-degrees Fahrenheit.
7. Bake the muffin cups for 15 minutes.
8. Evenly divide into suggested servings, let it cool, and store in meal prep ready container.

Nutrition Information:
Calories per serving: 310; Protein: 29.0g; Fat: 20.0g; Carbohydrates: 3.4g; Fiber: 0.4g

Ketogenic Quiche

Servings per Recipe: 6

Cooking Time: 30 minutes

Ingredients:

- 2 tsp dried thyme
- 1 tsp black pepper, ground
- 1 tsp salt
- 1 cup heavy cream
- 12 large eggs
- 1 large white onion, chopped
- 2 tbsp butter
- 2 cups Colby jack cheese, shredded

Directions:

1. In a skillet, add the butter and let it melt under medium low heat. Sauté the vegetables until the onion become translucent. Set aside to cool.
2. Crack the 12 eggs in a large mixing bowl and add the spices and cream. Beat together until the mixture becomes frothy. Set aside.
3. In a buttered quiche pan or deep pie pans, put 2 cups of shredded cheese as the first layer. Add ½ of the cooled vegetables and spread evenly on top of the cheese layer.
4. Add ½ of the egg mixture on top of the cheese and vegetable layer.
5. Continue piling up the layers. Spread the remaining cheese as the final layer of the quiche.
6. Bake the quiche for 20 to 25 minutes in a 350-degrees Fahrenheit pre-heated oven.
7. Use a knife or a fork and insert it in the middle of the pan. If it comes out clean, then the quiche is ready.
8. Evenly divide into suggested servings, let it cool, and store in meal prep ready container.

Nutrition Information:

Calories per serving: 406; Protein: 22.3g; Fat: 32.9g; Carbohydrates: 5.0g; Fiber: 0.6g

Ketogenic Fried Bacon and Eggs

Servings per Recipe: 4
Cooking Time: 25 minutes

Ingredients:
- ½ cup cheese, shredded
- 4 large eggs
- ½ of large white onion, chopped
- ½ cup celery, chopped
- ½ cup broccoli, chopped
- 1 carrot, peeled and chopped
- 8 bacon slices
- 1 tablespoon butter

Directions:
1. Put one tablespoon butter in a frying pan under medium heat.
2. Add the bacon and pan fry for 10 minutes or until crisped.
3. Add chopped vegetables and sauté 8 minutes or until the vegetables start to caramelize.
4. Spread the bacon and vegetable mixture evenly on the pan and free 4 empty spots in the pan where the eggs can go.
5. Break an egg on each free space created in the pan. Continue cooking until the yolks are done.
6. Evenly divide into suggested servings, let it cool, and store in meal prep ready container. Add shredded cheese once ready to eat.

Nutrition Information:
Calories per serving: 226; Protein: 16.0g; Fat: 16.1g; Carbohydrates: 4.0g; Fiber: 1g

Spinach and Egg-white Omelet

Servings per Recipe: 1
Cooking Time: 15 minutes

Ingredients:

- 1 clove garlic, minced
- Salt and pepper to taste
- Olive oil or cooking spray
- 1 tablespoon basil
- 1 whole red onion, chopped
- 1 handful shredded spinach
- 1 tomato, chopped
- 30ml almond milk
- 1 egg yolk
- 5 egg whites

Directions:

1. Spray a frying pan with cooking spray and place fire on medium heat.
2. Sauté the garlic, online and basil first until they become slightly golden brown. Add the spinach and let it wilt. Set aside the vegetable mixture.
3. Beat the egg yolk, egg whites and almond milk in a separate bowl.
4. Season with salt and pepper to taste. In an empty frying pan, spray the pan with oil and heat it under medium high heat.
5. Pour the egg and wait for it to get firm before putting the vegetables back. Fold the eggs to cover the vegetables and continue cooking for three to four minutes.
6. Evenly divide into suggested servings, let it cool, and store in meal prep ready container.

Nutrition Information:

Calories per serving: 249; Protein: 25.0g; Fat: 5.9g; Carbohydrates: 25.0g; Fiber: 4.7g

Feta-Kale Egg Casserole

Serves: 6

Cooking Time: 3 hours 4 minutes

Ingredients:

- Salt and pepper to taste
- 5-ounce baby kale
- ¼ cup sliced green onion
- 5-ounce crumbled Feta cheese
- 8 eggs
- 1 cup low-fat sour cream

Instructions:

1. Grease sides and bottom of Slow Cooker with cooking spray.
2. Place a nonstick skillet on medium high fire and grease with cooking spray.
3. Sauté kale until it is flat and softened, around 4 minutes.
4. In a large bowl, beat eggs and season with pepper and salt.
5. Mix in kale, green onion and feta cheese.
6. Pour into pot, cover, and cook on low for 3 hours.
7. Once done, evenly divide into suggested servings, let it cool, and store in meal prep ready container.
8. When ready to eat, place a dollop of sour cream on top of each serving.

Nutrition information:

Calories per serving: 331; Protein: 19.6g; Fat: 24.2g; Carbohydrates: 8.5g; Fiber: 1g

Cream Cheese & Mushroom Egg Casserole

Serves: 8

Cooking Time: 2 hours 40 minutes

Ingredients:
- Pepper and salt to taste
- 12 medium eggs
- ½ cup milk
- 8-ounce cream cheese, cut into small cubes
- 8-ounce fresh mushrooms, cleaned and sliced
- ½ cup shredded Mexican blend cheese

Instructions:
1. Grease sides and bottom of Slow Cooker with cooking spray.
2. Place a nonstick skillet on medium high fire and cook mushrooms for 10 minutes, until soft.
3. Meanwhile, whisk well eggs. Season with pepper and salt.
4. Pour in milk and whisk well.
5. With a slotted spoon, transfer softened mushrooms into slow cooker and evenly spread on the bottom.
6. Top with cream cheese.
7. Pour in egg mixture.
8. Top with cheese.
9. Cover and cook for 2.5 hours on high settings.
10. Evenly divide into suggested servings, let it cool, and store in meal prep ready container.

Nutrition information:
Calories per serving: 299; Protein: 15.3g; Fat: 17.2g; Carbohydrates: 24.2g; Fiber: 3.3g

Cauliflower Breakfast Quiche

Serves: 8
Cooking Time: 6 hours

Ingredients:
- Pepper and salt to taste
- 12 eggs
- ½ cup milk
- 2 cups cheese
- 1 head cauliflower, shredded
- 2 (5-ounce) packages of pre-cooked breakfast sausages, sliced

Instructions:
1. Grease sides and bottom of Slow Cooker with cooking spray.
2. In a large bowl, lightly beat eggs, pepper and salt.
3. Pour in milk and whisk well.
4. To assemble, place 1/3 of shredded cauliflower in bottom of cooker in an even layer, followed by 1/3 of the sliced sausages, and then 1/3 of the cheese. Season with pepper and salt.
5. Repeat this layering and seasoning process two more times.
6. Then pour in the egg mixture.
7. Cover and cook on low for 6 hours or until set and the sides are lightly browned.

Nutrition information:
Calories per serving: 481; Protein: 28.3g; Fat: 38.4g; Carbohydrates: 4.7g; Fiber: 0.7g

Breakfast Burger in Slow Cooker

Serves: 2

Cooking Time: 4 hours

Ingredients:
- Pepper and salt to taste
- 1 tablespoon butter
- 2 large eggs
- 2-ounce Pepper jack cheese
- 4-ounce sausage

Instructions:
1. Grease sides and bottom of Slow Cooker with cooking spray.
2. In a medium bowl, break the sausage, season with pepper and salt.
3. Mix well and knead with a fork.
4. Divide into two and form into a patty.
5. Divide butter into two pieces and place in slow cooker.
6. Add one patty on top of each butter.
7. Cover and cook on high for 3 hours.
8. Turnover patty, add cheese on top, and continue cooking for another hour.
9. Evenly divide into suggested servings, let it cool, and store in meal prep ready container.

Nutrition information:
Calories per serving: 366; Protein: 20.7g; Fat: 29.2g; Carbohydrates: 8.5g; Fiber: 1.9g

Baked Eggs Greek Style

Serves: 6
Cooking Time: 25 minutes

Ingredients:

- Pepper and salt to taste
- ½ tsp oregano
- ½ cup Feta cheese
- ¼ cup sun dried tomatoes
- 1 cup chopped kale
- 12 eggs

Instructions:

1. Grease a 9-inch round baking pan and preheat oven to 350°F.
2. In a large bowl, whisk eggs well. Season with pepper and salt.
3. Stir in oregano, cheese, dried tomatoes, and kale.
4. Pour into prepared pan and bake for 25 minutes.
5. Once done cooking, evenly divide into suggested servings, let it cool, and store in meal prep ready container.

Nutrition information:

Calories per serving: 175; Protein: 15.0g; Fat: 11.1g; Carbohydrates: 5.2g; Fiber: 1.5g

Egg and Sausage Sandwich

Serves: 2
Cooking Time: 10 minutes

Ingredients:

- 2 slices sharp cheddar cheese
- 2 sausage patties
- 1 tbsp mayonnaise
- 2 large eggs
- 1 tbsp butter

Instructions:

1. Cook the sausage patties according to manufacturer's instructions and keep warm.
2. Place a large skillet on medium fire and melt butter.
3. Using mason jar rings, place two of them in middle of pan.
4. Break the eggs in each ring and whisk a bit with your fork. Cover pan and let eggs cook for 6 to 8 minutes or until cooked through.
5. Transfer eggs to a plate. To assemble, place one egg, slather mayonnaise on egg, top with patties, and end with another egg on top.
6. Evenly divide in two, let it cool and store in meal prep ready container.

Nutrition information:

Calories per serving: 440; Protein: 16g; Fat: 41g; Carbohydrates: 4g; Fiber: 1g

Keto-Approved Breakfast Pizza

Serves: 8
Cooking Time: 30 minutes

Ingredients:
- 1 cup cheese, shredded
- 2 cups peppers, diced
- 8-oz sausage
- ¼ tsp pepper
- ½ tsp salt
- ½ cup heavy cream
- 12 eggs

Instructions:
1. Preheat oven to 350°F.
2. Place a cast-iron skillet on medium high fire and cook sausage until browned, around 6 minutes. Add peppers and cook for another 5 minutes.
3. Meanwhile, whisk well eggs in a large bowl. Season with pepper and salt. Whisk in cream.
4. Pour mixture into skillet and cook for 5 minutes and then transfer to the oven and bake for 15 minutes more.
5. Add cheese and broil for 3 minutes.
6. Let it cool, evenly divide into suggested servings, and store in meal prep ready container.

Nutrition information:
Calories per serving: 307; Protein: 18.4g; Fat: 24.3g; Carbohydrates: 2.6g; Fiber: 0.4g

Keto-Approved Pancakes

Serves: 4
Cooking Time: 16 minutes

Ingredients:
- 2-oz coconut oil
- 1 tbsp ground psyllium husk powder
- 7-oz cottage cheese
- 4 eggs
- 8 tbsp fresh blueberries
- 1 cup heavy whipping cream

Instructions:
1. In a medium bowl, whisk well eggs. Add psyllium powder and cheese. Mix well and let it stand for 10 minutes until thickened.
2. Place a nonstick skillet on medium fire and heat oil.
3. When skillet is hot, add ¼ of the batter. Cook for 3 minutes. Flip and cook for a minute.
4. Cook remaining batter.
5. Let it cool and store in meal prep ready container.
6. When ready to eat, whisk ¼ cup cream and place on top of 1 pancake with 2 tbsp blueberries.

Nutrition information:
Calories per serving: 425; Protein: 13g; Fat: 39g; Carbohydrates: 8g; Fiber: 3g

Keto-Approved Breakfast Porridge

Serves: 4
Cooking Time: 5 minutes

Ingredients:
- ¼ tsp salt
- 4 tbsp sunflower seeds
- 4 tbsp chia seeds
- 4 tbsp flaxseed, whole
- 4 cup unsweetened almond milk

Instructions:
1. In a medium pot, mix all ingredients and bring to a simmer.
2. Simmer for 5 minutes or until thickened.
3. Turn off fire and let it cool.
4. Evenly divide into suggested servings, store in mason jars and refrigerate.

Nutrition information:
Calories per serving: 261; Protein: 14.4g; Fat: 13.6g; Carbohydrates: 22.7g; Fiber: 8.4g

Bacon and Cheese Stuffed Peppers

Serves: 6
Cooking Time: 12 minutes

Ingredients:
- 1 tsp Worcestershire sauce
- ½ cup shredded cheddar cheese
- ½ tsp garlic powder
- 4 slices bacon, cooked and crumbled
- 2 tbsp green onions, sliced
- 4-oz cream cheese
- 6 mini sweet peppers

Instructions:
1. Lightly grease a cooking sheet with cooking spray and preheat oven to 400°F.
2. Divide the mini peppers in half. Deseed, remove the inner membranes and set aside.
3. With a mixer, mix well in a medium bowl the rest of the ingredients.
4. Spoon the mixture into the pepper cavity. Place the stuffed peppers on prepared sheet.
5. Pop in the oven and bake for 11 minutes or until cheese is melted.
6. Let it cool, evenly divide into suggested servings, and store in meal prep ready container.

Nutrition information:
Calories per serving: 174; Protein: 2g; Fat: 7g; Carbohydrates: 1g; Fiber: 0.5g

Keto Meal-Prep Lunch/Dinner Recipes

Slow Cooked Corned Beef

Serves: 6

Cooking Time: 9 hours

Ingredients:

- 2 cups water
- 2-pounds corned beef brisket with seasoning packet
- 1 cabbage, cut into wedges
- 2 onions, chopped

Instructions:

1. In cold running water, rinse corned beef and then dry with paper towels.
2. Place corned beef in slow cooker and sprinkle seasoning packet.
3. Add onions, cabbage, and water.
4. Cover and cook on low for 9 hours.
5. Let it cool, evenly divide into suggested servings, and store in meal prep ready container.

Nutrition information:

Calories per serving: 314; Protein: 22.6g; Fat: 22.6g; Carbohydrates: 3.6g; Fiber: 0.6g

Beef Brisket with Cranberry Gravy

Serves: 7

Cooking Time: 8 hours

Ingredients:
- ½ teaspoon salt
- ¼ teaspoon pepper
- ½ cup chopped onion
- 1 (8-ounce) can tomato sauce
- 1 (14-ounce) whole-berry cranberry sauce
- 1 fresh beef brisket (2 ½-pounds)
- 1 tablespoon prepared mustard

Instructions:
1. Chop beef into 1-inch cubes and spread on bottom of slow cooker.
2. Add remaining ingredients into pot.
3. Cover and cook on low for 8 hours.
4. Let it cool, evenly divide into suggested servings, and store in meal prep ready container.

Nutrition information:
Calories per serving: 264; Protein: 24.9g; Fat: 24.4g; Carbohydrates: 29.7g; Fiber: 2.7g

Keto Swiss Steak

Serves: 6
Cooking Time: 8 hours

Ingredients:
- ¼ teaspoon pepper
- ½ teaspoon salt
- 1 ½-pounds beef round steak, cut into 6 pieces
- 1 celery rib, cut into ½-inch slices
- 1 medium onion, sliced into ¼-inch pieces
- 2 (8-ounce) cans tomato sauce

Instructions:
1. Add all ingredients in slow cooker.
2. Mix well.
3. Cover and cook for 8 hours on low.
4. Let it cool, evenly divide into suggested servings, and store in meal prep ready container.

Nutrition information:
Calories per serving: 236; Protein: 27.3g; Fat: 4.6g; Carbohydrates: 17.3g; Fiber: 4.6g

Baked Herbed Salmon

Serves: 4
Cooking Time: 15 minutes

Ingredients:
- ¼ tsp tarragon
- ¼ tsp thyme
- ½ cup soy sauce
- ½ tsp basil
- ½ tsp ground ginger
- ½ tsp rosemary
- 1 tsp minced garlic
- 1 tsp oregano leaves
- 2 pounds salmon fillet
- 1 tbsp sesame oil

Instructions:
1. In a Ziploc back, place the sesame oil, soy sauce and spices and shake thoroughly until well combined. Put the salmon pieces in the Ziploc bag. Refrigerate the salmon with the marinade for 4 hours.
2. Preheat the oven to 350°F. Place the marinated salmon on a baking pan lined with aluminum foil.
3. Bake the marinated salmon for 15 minutes.
4. Let it cool, evenly divide into suggested servings, and store in meal prep ready container.

Nutrition information:
Calories per serving: 448; Protein: 50.7g; Fat: 21.9g; Carbohydrates: 8.6g; Fiber: 0.9g

Ginger Beef Asian Style

Serves: 2

Cooking Time: 25 minutes

Ingredients:
- Salt and pepper to taste
- 4 tbsp apple cider vinegar
- 1 tsp ground ginger
- 2 small tomatoes, diced
- 1 crushed garlic clove
- 1 diced small onion
- 1 tbsp olive oil
- 2 sirloin steaks at 4oz each, cut into strips
- Cooking spray

Instructions:
1. Lightly grease large skillet with cooking spray and heat under medium-high fire.
2. Add the steaks and sear for 2 minutes per side.
3. Add the garlic, onion and tomatoes. Cook for 3 minutes.
4. In a separate bowl, add the salt, pepper, ginger and vinegar.
5. Mix well before adding the mixture into the skillet.
6. Mix and cover the skillet.
7. Turn the heat to low and simmer until the liquid is reduced completely, around 15 minutes.
8. Let it cool, evenly divide into suggested servings, and store in meal prep ready container.

Nutrition information:

Calories per serving: 345; Protein: 25.3g; Fat: 22.0g; Carbohydrates: 10.4g; Fiber: 2.2g

Asian-Inspired Keto Pork Chops

Serves: 4
Cooking Time: 20 minutes

Ingredients:
- ½ tbsp Sambal chili paste
- ½ tbsp sugar-free ketchup
- ½ tsp five spice powder
- ½ tsp pepper corn
- 1 ½ tsp soy sauce
- 1 medium star anise
- 1 stalk lemongrass
- 1 tbsp almond flour
- 1 tbsp fish sauce
- 1 tsp Sesame oil
- 4 boneless pork chops
- 4 halved garlic cloves, crushed

Instructions:
1. Place the pork chops on a stable working surface. With a rolling pin wrapped in wax paper, pound the pork chop to ½ inch thickness.
2. In a blender, puree star anise, pepper corns, lemon grass, and garlic.
3. Add soy sauce, fish sauce, five spice powder and sesame oil. Mix well. This will be the marinade.
4. Put the pork chops in a baking tray and add marinade. Toss or massage the marinade into the pork chops. Let it sit for 2 hours at room temperature.
5. Heat skillet and add a little amount oil for frying.
6. Separately, coat the pork chops with almond flour. Put the pork chops in the pan and sear 3 minutes per side.
7. Cook for two minutes each side until it becomes golden brown in color.
8. Mix sugar-free ketchup and sambal chili paste to make a sauce.
9. Let it cool, evenly divide into suggested servings, and store in meal prep ready container. Serve sauce on the side when ready to enjoy.

Nutrition information:
Calories per serving: 266; Protein: 42.5g; Fat: 8.2g; Carbohydrates: 3.0g; Fiber: 0.6g

Ground Beef and Cabbage Stir-Fry

Serves: 5

Cooking Time: 20 minutes

Ingredients:

- ¼ teaspoon ground black pepper
- 1 1⁄3-lbs ground beef
- 1 2⁄3-lbs green cabbage, shredded
- 1 tablespoon fresh ginger, finely chopped or grated
- 1 teaspoon sesame oil
- 1 tablespoon white wine vinegar
- 1 teaspoon chili flakes
- 1 teaspoon onion powder
- 1 teaspoon salt
- 2 garlic cloves
- 3 scallions, in slices
- 3 tablespoons butter

Instructions:

1. In a large pan melt 2 tbsps. of the butter. Add shredded cabbage and stir fry for 4 minutes.
2. Stir in pepper, vinegar, onion powder, and salt. Continue stir frying for another 3 minutes. When wilted, transfer to a bowl and set aside.
3. In same pan, heat remaining butter and sauté ginger, chili flakes, and garlic for two minutes.
4. Stir in ground beef and cook for 8 minutes until no longer pink.
5. Stir in cabbage and scallions. Add sesame oil and cook for 3 minutes.
6. Let it cool, evenly divide into suggested servings, and store in meal prep ready container.

Nutrition information:

Calories per serving: 392; Protein: 36.7g; Fat: 22.6g; Carbohydrates: 10.4g; Fiber: 3.5g

Chicken Marsala Casserole

Serves: 4
Cooking Time: 25 minutes

Ingredients:
- 1 red bell pepper, finely diced
- 1 tablespoon fresh parsley, finely chopped
- 1 tsp salt
- 1¼ cups coconut cream or heavy whipping cream
- 1½-lbs chicken breasts
- 2 ½ tablespoons garam masala
- 3 tablespoons butter

Instructions:
1. Preheat oven to 400°F.
2. Place a large cast iron pan on medium high fire and melt butter.
3. Slice chicken breasts lengthwise and pan fry for 3 minutes per side.
4. Add 1 tablespoon of garam masala to pan and stir fry chicken for 2 minutes.
5. Turn off fire. Season chicken with salt. Add remaining ingredients in pan and mix well.
6. Pop in the oven and bake for 20 minutes.
7. Let it cool, evenly divide into suggested servings, and store in meal prep ready container.

Nutrition information:
Calories per serving: 629; Protein: 38g.0; Fat: 51.0g; Carbohydrates: 10g; Fiber: 4g

Traditional Filipino Adobo

Serves: 4
Cooking Time: 35 minutes

Ingredients:
- ¼ cup vinegar
- ¼ cup water
- ½ cup soy sauce
- 1 bay leaf
- 1 medium onion, chopped
- 1 tablespoon coconut oil
- 1 tablespoon whole peppercorns
- 4 garlic cloves, smashed and chopped roughly with skin
- 4-pieces chicken legs, skinless and cut into thigh and drumstick pieces

Instructions:
1. In a medium pot, add oil, and heat over medium high fire.
2. Once hot, sauté garlic for 2 minutes or until browned.
3. Add onions and sauté until soft and translucent, around 5 minutes.
4. Add chicken and peppercorn. Brown for 3 minutes per side.
5. Add soy sauce, peppercorns, vinegar, bay leaf, and water.
6. Bring to a simmer, lower fire to medium, and cover.
7. Cook for 15 minutes. Uncover and increase fire to medium high.
8. Continue cooking for 5 minutes or until more than half of the sauce has evaporated.
9. Let it cool, evenly divide into suggested servings, and store in meal prep ready container.

Nutrition information:
Calories per serving: 293; Protein: 35.7g; Fat: 13.2g; Carbohydrates: 7.0g; Fiber: 1.3g

Pesto Chicken Casserole

Serves: 5
Cooking Time: 30 minutes

Ingredients:
- ½-pound feta cheese, diced
- 1 2/3 cups heavy whipping cream
- 1 garlic clove, chopped finely
- 1 tablespoon butter
- 1.5-pounds chicken breasts
- 3.5-ounce green pesto
- 8 tablespoons pitted olive
- Pepper and salt to taste

Instructions:
1. Preheat oven to 400°F.
2. Slice chicken breast into 1-inch cubes. Season with pepper and salt.
3. In a large cast-iron pot, heat butter over medium high flame.
4. Add garlic and sauté until browned, around 3 minutes.
5. Add sliced chicken and cook until no longer pink, around 8 minutes.
6. Stir in feta cheese, olives, whipping cream, and green pesto. Stir well.
7. Pop in the oven and bake for 20 minutes.
8. Let it cool, evenly divide into suggested servings, and store in meal prep ready container.

Nutrition information:
Calories per serving: 533.6; Protein: 36.0g; Fat: 40.9g; Carbohydrates: 4.9g; Fiber: 0.8g

Goat Curry Mediterranean Style

Serves: 4
Cooking Time: 65 minutes

Ingredients:

- ½ cup water
- ½ pound potatoes
- 1 ½ inch knob fresh ginger
- 1 bay leaf
- 1 tablespoon coriander powder
- 1 teaspoon cumin powder
- 1 teaspoon garam masala
- 1 teaspoon Kashmiri chili powder
- 1 teaspoon paprika
- 1 teaspoon turmeric powder
- 2 (14 ounce) cans organic diced tomatoes
- 2 onions, chopped
- 2 pounds goat meat
- 2 tablespoons avocado oil
- 2 teaspoons salt
- 3 cloves garlic, peeled, smashed, and chopped
- 4 cardamom pods
- 4 cloves

Instructions:

1. Press sauté button on Instant Pot or pressure cooker, and heat oil.
2. Once oil is hot, brown goat meat for 10 minutes.
3. Add garlic, ginger, and onions. Sauté for 5 minutes.
4. Stir in paprika, Kashmiri, turmeric, salt, cumin, coriander, cardamom pods, cloves, garam masala, and bay leaf. Sauté for 2 minutes.
5. Add potatoes, water, and diced tomatoes. Mix well.
6. Cover, press cancel button, press meat/stew button, and increase time to 45 minutes.
7. Do a natural release method.
8. Let it cool, evenly divide into suggested servings, and store in meal prep ready container.

Nutrition information:

Calories per serving: 477; Protein: 64.6g; Fat: 14.5g; Carbohydrates: 20.0g; Fiber: 3.6g

Slow-Cooked Beef Moroccan Style

Serves: 8
Cooking Time: 8 hours

Ingredients:
- ½ cup apricots
- ½ cup sliced yellow onions
- 1 teaspoon sea salt
- 2 cups water
- 2 pounds beef roast
- 4 tablespoons garam masala seasoning

Instructions:
1. Place onions and apricots on bottom of Instant Pot.
2. Rub salt and garam masala all over roast beef and place roast beef on top of onions and apricots.
3. Pour water.
4. Cover, press slow cook button, adjust cooking time to 6 hours.
5. Once done cooking, remove roast beef and shred with 2 forks.
6. Return to pot, cover, press slow cook and adjust time to 2 hours.
7. Let it cool, evenly divide into suggested servings, and store in meal prep ready container.

Nutrition information:
Calories per serving: 275; Protein: 31.9g; Fat: 14.7g; Carbohydrates: 3.0g; Fiber: 0.7g

Beef Stroganoff Keto Style

Serves: 8
Cooking Time: 20 minutes

Ingredients:
- ½ pound blue cheese
- ½ pound mushrooms
- ½ teaspoon salt
- 1 ½ cups sour cream
- 1 pinch ground black pepper
- 1 tablespoon dried thyme
- 1 yellow onion, chopped
- 1-pound ground beef
- 4 zucchinis, peeled and spiralized
- 3 tablespoons butter

Instructions:
1. In medium pot over medium high fire, melt butter.
2. Once butter is melted, stir in onions and sauté until soft and translucent, around 4 minutes.
3. Add beef and sauté for 7 minutes. Season with salt and pepper.
4. Stir in sour cream blue cheese, and thyme.
5. Bring to a simmer. Lower fire to medium low. Cover and cook for 15 minutes.
6. Meanwhile, evenly divide spiralized zucchini into four meal prep containers.
7. Once stroganoff mixture has cooled, top each spiralized zucchini with 1/8 of the stroganoff mixture and store.

Nutrition information:
Calories per serving: 363; Protein: 23.0g; Fat: 27.5g; Carbohydrates: 5.9g; Fiber: 0.6g

Baked Cod Topped with Arugula Tapenade

Serves: 2

Cooking Time: 10 minutes

Ingredients:

- ½ cup pitted black olives
- 1 medium lemon
- 1-pound cod fillet
- 2 tablespoons capers, rinsed medium garlic clove, chopped roughly
- 3 cups arugula
- Pepper and salt to taste

Instructions:

1. Preheat oven to 400°F.
2. Slice the lemon into ¼-inch thick circles and layer at the bottom of a small baking dish.
3. Season cod with pepper and salt, generously.
4. Place fish on top of lemon slices.
5. When ready, pop fish in oven and bake for 10 minutes.
6. Meanwhile, in a blender or food processor, process the tapenade by adding the garlic, capers, olives, and arugula. Pulse until roughly chopped and resembles a tapenade.
7. Let it cool, evenly divide into suggested servings, place in meal prep ready container, top with tapenade, and store.

Nutrition information:

Calories per serving: 216; Protein: 36.4g; Fat: 4.5g; Carbohydrates: 7.3g; Fiber: 2.2g

Baked Salmon Topped with Caper-Relish

Serves: 4
Cooking Time: 12 minutes

Ingredients:
- 1 tablespoon extra-virgin olive oil
- 1 tablespoon cider vinegar
- 2 tablespoons capers, rinsed and minced
- 1 shallot, minced
- Pepper and salt to taste
- 4 6-ounce fillets of salmon
- 2 tablespoons minced fresh tarragon, stems reserved
- 2 tablespoons minced fresh parsley, stems reserved
- 1 lemon, sliced into ¼-inch thick circles

Instructions:
1. Preheat oven to 400°F and lightly grease a 9x13-inch baking dish.
2. Place lemon slices on bottom of prepared dish and scatter herb stems on top of lemon.
3. Season salmon with pepper and salt. Then, place salmon on top of lemon slices with skin side down and touching the lemons.
4. When ready, pop in the oven and bake for 12 minutes.
5. Meanwhile, make the relish by mixing in a small bowl the olive oil, vinegar, capers, shallot, tarragon, and parsley. Season with pepper and salt to taste.
6. Let salmon cool, evenly divide into suggested servings, place in meal prep ready containers, top each salmon with ¼ of the caper relish, and store.

Nutrition information:
Calories per serving: 288; Protein: 37.2g; Fat: 13.6g; Carbohydrates: 2.1g; Fiber: 0.4g

Chicken in Coco-Turmeric Sauce

Serves: 8

Cooking Time: 40 minutes

Ingredients:

- ½ cup coconut milk, unsweetened
- 1 whole chicken, cut into pieces
- 2 inch-knob fresh ginger, grated
- 2 inch-knob fresh turmeric, grated
- 4 cloves of garlic, grated
- Salt and pepper to taste
- 1 tbsp oil
- 1 stalk lemongrass, folded and tied
- 1 ½ cups water

Instructions:

1. In a medium pot on medium high fire heat oil.
2. Add chicken and brown for 5 minutes per side. Remove from pot and set aside.
3. In same pot, add garlic sauté for a minute. Add ginger and sauté for another minute.
4. Stir in turmeric and lemongrass. Cook for a minute.
5. Return chicken and sauté in mixture for 3 minutes. Season generously with pepper and salt.
6. Add water, cover, and bring to a simmer. Lower fire to medium and simmer for 15 minutes.
7. Add coconut milk and cook until heated through, around 3 minutes.
8. Adjust seasoning to taste.
9. Let it cool, evenly divide into suggested servings, and store in meal prep ready container.

Nutrition information:

Calories per serving: 270; Protein: 24.5g; Fat: 18.9g; Carbohydrates: 4.2g; Fiber: 1.6g

Fajita Chicken

Serves: 8

Cooking Time: 60 minutes

Ingredients:

- ½ teaspoon chipotle pepper, chopped
- ½ teaspoon cumin
- 1 cup roma tomatoes, diced
- 1 onion, sliced
- 1 teaspoon ground coriander
- 2 ½ pounds chicken thighs and breasts, skin and bones removed
- 2 cups bell peppers, sliced
- 4 cloves of garlic, minced
- Salt and pepper to taste

Instructions:

1. In a large pot, add oil and heat over medium-high fire.
2. Add chicken and brown for 5 minutes per side. Remove from pot and transfer to a plate.
3. In same pot, sauté garlic for a minute. Add onions and sauté for 4 minutes. Add tomatoes, pepper, and cumin. Cook for 5 minutes more.
4. Return chicken to pot and mix well. Sauté for 5 minutes.
5. Season with pepper and salt. Add bell pepper and water.
6. Cover, bring to a simmer, and simmer for 15 minutes.
7. Remove chicken and shred with two forks. Return to pot and adjust seasoning.
8. If desired, continue cooking until sauce has evaporated to desired level.
9. Let it cool, evenly divide into suggested servings, and store in meal prep ready container.

Nutrition information:

Calories per serving: 328; Protein: 39.5g; Fat: 17.7g; Carbohydrates: 3.3g; Fiber: 1.7g

Creamy Crab-Spinach Bake

Serves: 3
Cooking Time: 40 minutes

Ingredients:
- ½ cup heavy cream
- ½ cup water
- ½ tsp minced garlic
- 1 tbs flour
- 10-oz box of frozen spinach
- 2 tbsp shredded Parmesan
- 2 tbsp unsalted butter
- 2 tbsp white wine
- 8-oz crab meat
- salt and pepper

Instructions:
1. Lightly grease a small baking dish with cooking spray and preheat oven to 350°F.
2. Thoroughly drain spinach and spread on bottom of baking dish.
3. In a small pot on medium fire, melt butter. Add garlic and flour. Stir well and cook for 2 minutes. Stir in wine, water, and cream. Cook while stirring constantly until mixture has thickened, around 5 minutes.
4. Stir in crab and parmesan in pot. Add seasoning to taste and mix well.
5. Pour mixture on top of spinach and bake in the oven for 25 minutes.
6. Let it cool, evenly divide into suggested servings, and store in meal prep ready container.

Nutrition information:
Calories per serving: 326.7; Protein: 19.3g; Fat: 24g; Carbohydrates: 7.3g; Fiber: 2.7g

Ground Beef and Cheese Casserole

Serves: 8
Cooking Time: 60 minutes

Ingredients:

- ½-pound bacon, diced
- 1 clove garlic
- 1 tablespoon Worcestershire sauce
- 1 tablespoon yellow mustard
- 1 teaspoon fresh dill
- 1 teaspoon ground pepper
- 1 teaspoon hot sauce
- 1 teaspoon seasoned salt
- 1/2 sweet onion
- 1/4 cup heavy cream
- 1-pound ground beef
- 2 tablespoons reduced sugar ketchup
- 4 large eggs
- 4 tablespoons cream cheese
- 8-ounces grated cheddar

Instructions:

1. Lightly grease an 8x8-inch baking dish and preheat oven to 350°F.
2. On medium high fire, cook bacon to a crisped in a large cast-iron skillet. Once done cooking, transfer to a plate and drain fat.
3. In same skillet, brown ground beef for 10 minutes. Once done cooking drain fat.
4. Add garlic and onions to beef and cook for 5 minutes.
5. Stir in seasoned salt, Worcestershire sauce, mustard, ketchup, and cream cheese. Sauté for 5 minutes. Then spread on bottom of baking dish.

6. Spread bacon on top of ground beef.
7. In a medium bowl, whisk well the eggs. Stir in heavy cream, hot sauce, and pepper. Whisk thoroughly. Pour over ground beef.
8. Top mixture with cheese and pop in the oven. Bake until tops are golden, around 30 minutes.
9. Once done cooking, remove from oven and sprinkle dill on top.
10. Let it cool, evenly divide into suggested servings, and store in meal prep ready container.

Nutrition information:

Calories per serving: 436.5; Protein: 32.2g; Fat: 32.2g; Carbohydrates: 1.5g; Fiber: 0g

Zucchini and Cheese Gratin

Serves: 9
Cooking Time: 45 minutes

Ingredients:
- 1 1/2 cups shredded pepper jack cheese
- 1 small onion, peeled and sliced thin
- 1/2 cup heavy whipping cream
- 1/2 tsp garlic powder
- 2 Tbsp butter
- 4 cups raw zucchini, sliced into ¼-inch thin circles
- salt and pepper to taste

Instructions:
1. Lightly grease a 9x9-inch baking dish and preheat oven to 375°F.
2. In dish, overlap 1/3 of onion and zucchini slices. Season with pepper and salt and sprinkle ½ of cheese on top.
3. Repeat layering two more times with no cheese on top of the last layer.
4. Meanwhile, in a microwave safe bowl, whisk well heavy cream, butter, and garlic powder. Melt in the microwave for a minute and mix well. If needed, heat some more to mix thoroughly.
5. Pour over dish. Pop in the oven and bake until tops are golden brown, around 45 minutes.
6. Let it cool, evenly divide into suggested servings, and store in meal prep ready container.

Nutrition information:
Calories per serving: 280; Protein: 8g; Fat: 20g; Carbohydrates: 5g; Fiber: 2g

Vegetable-Chicken Creamy Casserole

Serves: 8

Cooking Time: 30 minutes

Ingredients:

- 1 1/2 Cups Shredded Cheddar Cheese
- 1 8-ounce Cream Cheese Softened
- 1 Cup Cottage Cheese pureed in a blender - see note below
- 1 Medium Zucchini Diced
- 1 Small/Medium Yellow Squash Diced
- 1 Teaspoon Garlic Powder
- 1 Teaspoon Mineral Salt
- 1 Teaspoon Onion Powder
- 1/2 Cup Grated Parmesan Cheese the green can kind is fine
- 1/2 Cup Sour Cream
- 1/4 Small Onion Diced (Optional)
- 2 Cups Frozen Spinach
- 3 Cups Cooked Chicken Breast Diced or Shredded

Instructions:

1. Lightly grease with cooking spray a 9x13-inch baking dish and preheat oven to 350°F.
2. Except for ½ cup of shredded cheddar cheese, mix well all ingredients in a large bowl.
3. Pour evenly in prepared dish.
4. Sprinkle remaining cheese on top of casserole.
5. Bake in the oven until bubbly, around 30 minutes.
6. Let it cool, evenly divide into suggested servings, and store in meal prep ready container.

Nutrition information:

Calories per serving: 362.2; Protein: 30.1g; Fat: 23.4g; Carbohydrates: 8.2g; Fiber: 1.4g

Easy Meatballs

Serves: 6
Cooking Time: 25 minutes

Ingredients:
- 2 tablespoons olive oil
- 2 pounds ground beef
- 1 tablespoon cumin
- 1 teaspoon paprika
- 2 eggs, beaten
- 3 cloves of garlic, minced
- 1 tablespoon dried parsley
- Salt and pepper to taste

Instructions:
1. Lightly grease with cooking spray a baking sheet and preheat oven to 350°F.
2. Place all ingredients in the mixing bowl.
3. Form small balls using your hands and place ½-inch apart on prepared sheet.
4. Once done, pop in the oven and bake for 20 to 25 minutes.
5. Let it cool, evenly divide into suggested servings, and store in meal prep ready container.

Nutrition information:
Calories per serving: 413; Protein: 46.7g; Fat: 21.4g; Carbohydrates: 2.5g; Fiber: 0.9g

Slow Cooked Pork Carnitas

Serves: 12

Cooking Time: 12 hours

Ingredients:
- ½ cup lemon juice, freshly squeezed
- ½ cup lime juice, freshly squeezed
- ½ tablespoon salt
- 1 tablespoon garlic powder
- 1 tablespoon ground cumin
- 1 teaspoon black pepper
- 1 teaspoon cayenne pepper
- 1 teaspoon ground coriander
- 4 pounds pork shoulder

Instructions:
1. In slow cooker, except for pork shoulder add and mix all ingredients. Add pork shoulder and cover well with sauce.
2. Cover and cook on low for 12 hours or on high for 9 hours.
3. When done cooking, shred pork with two forks.
4. Let it cool, evenly divide into suggested servings, and store in meal prep ready container.

Nutrition information:
Calories per serving: 414; Protein: 38.3g; Fat: 29.6g; Carbohydrates: 2.8g; Fiber: 1.6g

Pork Ribs in Slow Cooker

Serves: 8
Cooking Time: 12 hours

Ingredients:
- ¾ teaspoon garlic powder
- 1 jalapeno pepper, cut into rings
- 1 tablespoon organic tomato paste
- 2 tablespoons coconut aminos
- 2 tablespoons rice vinegar
- 2 teaspoons Chinese five-spice powder
- 4 pounds baby back ribs
- Salt and pepper to taste

Instructions:
1. Mix all ingredients in slow cooker except for the ribs.
2. Add ribs and cover well with sauce.
3. Cover and cook on low for 12 hours or on high for 9 hours.
4. Let it cool, evenly divide into suggested servings, and store in meal prep ready container.

Nutrition information:
Calories per serving: 508; Protein: 45g; Fat: 35.7g; Carbohydrates: 1.8g; Fiber: 0.7g

Malaysian Style Beef Stew

Serves: 8
Cooking Time: 60 minutes

Ingredients:

- ½ cup cilantro leaves, chopped
- ½ cup desiccated coconut, toasted
- 1 beef shoulder
- 1 cup coconut cream
- 1 cup water
- 1 tablespoon coconut oil
- 1 teaspoon ground cumin
- 1 teaspoon salt
- 1 teaspoon turmeric powder
- 2 stalks lemon grass
- 2 teaspoon ground coriander
- 6 cloves of garlic, minced
- 6 dried birds eye chilies, chopped
- 6 kaffir lime leaves

Instructions:

1. In a large heavy-bottomed pot ass oil and heat over medium-high fire.
2. Once oil is hot, add beef shoulder and brown for 5 minutes per side. When done browning, transfer to a chopping board and cut into 1-inch cubes.
3. Meanwhile, in same pot add garlic and sauté for a minute. Stir in desiccated coconut, chilies, cumin, coriander, turmeric, lime leaves, and lemongrass. Sauté for 2 minutes.
4. Return chopped beef to pot and mix well.
5. Season with salt and add a cup of water. Bring to a simmer, lower fire to medium, cover, and simmer for 30 minutes.
6. Stir in coconut cream and cilantro leaves. Cover and cook for another 15 minutes or until beef is tender.
7. Let it cool, evenly divide into suggested servings, and store in meal prep ready container.

Nutrition information:

Calories per serving: 305; Protein: 32.3g; Fat: 18.7g; Carbohydrates: 6.5g; Fiber: 3.7g

Stir-Fried Mushrooms and Beef

Serves: 4

Cooking Time: 10 minutes

Ingredients:

- 2 tablespoons olive oil
- 2 tablespoons butter
- 2 cloves of garlic, minced
- 4 beef steaks, cut into strips (around 1.5-2 lbs)
- 2 cups mushrooms, sliced
- ½ tbsp oyster sauce
- ¼ tsp salt

Instructions:

1. Place a wok or a frying pan on high fire and let pan heat for a minute. Add oil and continue heating it for a minute or two until smoking.
2. Add garlic and mushrooms. Stir fry for two minutes.
3. Add beef and stir fry for 3 minutes.
4. Add butter, oyster sauce, and salt.
5. Mix well and stir fry for another minute.
6. Let it cool, evenly divide into suggested servings, and store in meal prep ready container.

Nutrition information:

Calories per serving: 440; Protein:35.2 g; Fat: 30.3g; Carbohydrates: 0.6g; Fiber: 0.2g

Beef Steak Filipino Style

Serves: 6
Cooking Time: 25 minutes

Ingredients:
- 2 tablespoons coconut oil
- 1 onion, sliced
- 4 beef steaks
- 3 tablespoons coconut aminos
- 2 tablespoons lemon juice, freshly squeezed

Instructions:
1. In nonstick fry pan, heat oil on medium high fire.
2. Pan fry beef steaks and season with coconut aminos.
3. Cook until dark brown, around 7 minutes per side. Transfer to a plate.
4. Sauté onions in same pan until caramelized, around 8 minutes. Season with lemon juice and return steaks in pan. Mix well.
5. Let it cool, evenly divide into suggested servings, and store in meal prep ready container.

Nutrition information:
Calories per serving: 260; Protein: 25.3g; Fat: 27.1g; Carbohydrates: 0.7g; Fiber: 0.3g

Pork Chops with Rosemary-Garlic Blend

Serves: 4
Cooking Time: 20 minutes

Ingredients:
- 1 tbsp freshly minced rosemary
- 1 tbsp olive oil
- 1/2 cup butter, melted
- 2 cloves garlic, minced
- 4 pork loin chops
- Freshly ground black pepper
- kosher salt

Instructions:
1. Preheat oven to 375°F.
2. Place a cast-iron skillet on medium high fire and heat oil.
3. Season porkchops with pepper and salt. Brown in skillet for 4 minutes per side.
4. Meanwhile, in a small bowl mix well garlic, rosemary, and butter.
5. Once chops are done browning, slather with the garlic-rosemary mixture.
6. Pop in the oven and bake for 12 minutes.
7. Let it cool, evenly divide into suggested servings, and store in meal prep ready container.

Nutrition information:
Calories per serving: 566; Protein: 40.6g; Fat: 43.8g; Carbohydrates: 1.0g; Fiber: 0.2g

Herbed-Crusted Baked Salmon

Serves: 4
Cooking Time: 7 minutes

Ingredients:
- 1 tbsp finely minced shallots
- 1 tbsp Grainy mustard
- 2 cloves garlic, finely minced
- 2 tsp fresh rosemary, chopped
- 2 tsp fresh thyme leaves, chopped, plus more for garnish
- 4 4-oz salmon fillets
- Freshly ground black pepper
- Juice of 1/2 lemon
- kosher salt
- Lemon slices, for serving

Instructions:
1. Line a baking sheet with foil and lightly grease with cooking spray.
2. Preheat oven to broil.
3. Evenly spread salmon prepared sheet and generously season with salt and pepper.
4. In a small bowl, whisk well lemon juice, rosemary, thyme, shallot, garlic, and mustard.
5. Pop in the oven and broil for 7 minutes.
6. Remove from oven and garnish with lemon slices and rosemary.
7. Let it cool, evenly divide into suggested servings, and store in meal prep ready container.

Nutrition information:
Calories per serving: 156; Protein: 23.7g; Fat: 5.2g; Carbohydrates: 2.7g; Fiber: 0.5g

Creamy Chicken Tuscan Style

Serves: 4

Cooking Time: 45 minutes

Ingredients:

- 1 1/2 cups cherry tomatoes
- 1 tbsp extra-virgin olive oil
- 1 tsp dried oregano
- 1/2 cup heavy cream
- 1/4 cup freshly grated Parmesan
- 2 cups baby spinach
- 3 cloves garlic, minced
- 3 tbsp unsalted butter
- 4 boneless skinless chicken breasts
- Freshly ground black pepper
- Kosher salt
- Lemon wedges, for serving

Instructions:

1. Place a large pan on medium high fire and add oil.
2. Season chicken with oregano, pepper, and salt.
3. Once hot, brown chicken for 8 minutes per side. Transfer to a plate.
4. In same pan, melt butter and cook garlic for a minute.
5. Stir in tomatoes. Season with pepper and salt. Cook for 5 minutes or until tomatoes start to burst and then add spinach. Cook for a minute.
6. Add parmesan and heavy cream. Bring to a simmer and reduce heat to medium and continue cooking for 5 minutes or until sauce has reduced slightly.
7. Return chicken and continue simmering for 7 minutes.
8. Let it cool, evenly divide into suggested servings, and store in meal prep ready container.
9. When ready to eat, squeeze lemon on chicken and enjoy.

Nutrition information:

Calories per serving: 507; Protein: 65.3g; Fat: 20.4g; Carbohydrates: 13.2g; Fiber: 1.7g

Tender Jerk Chicken

Serves: 6

Cooking Time: 35 minutes

Ingredients:

- 1 ½ pounds chicken drumstick, skin-on and bones removed
- 1 tsp nutmeg
- 1 tsp cinnamon
- 1 tsp all spice
- 1 tsp onion powder
- 1 thumb-size ginger, sliced
- 3 tablespoons extra-virgin olive oil
- Salt and pepper to taste
- 1 cup water

Instructions:

1. Place a medium pot on medium high fire and heat oil.
2. Once hot, brown chicken for 5 minutes per side.
3. Stir in nutmeg, cinnamon, all spice, onion powder, and ginger. Sauté for a minute.
4. Season with pepper and salt.
5. Add water. Cover, bring to a simmer, lower fir to medium, continue cooking for 20 minutes or until chicken is fork tender and liquid has evaporated.
6. Let it cool, evenly divide into suggested servings, and store in meal prep ready container.

Nutrition information:

Calories per serving: 217; Protein: 13.4g; Fat: 20.9g; Carbohydrates: 1.9g; Fiber: 1.3g

Buttered Chicken from India

Serves: 5
Cooking Time: 45 minutes

Ingredients:
- ½ teaspoon cayenne pepper
- 1 ½ teaspoons salt
- 1 can light coconut milk
- 1 can tomato paste
- 5 tbsp butter
- 1 tablespoon paprika
- 1 teaspoon cumin powder
- 1 teaspoon dried coriander
- 1 teaspoon turmeric powder
- 2 teaspoons garam masala
- 2-pounds boneless chicken breasts
- 9 cloves of garlic, crushed

Instructions:
1. Place a large pot on medium high fire and melt 3 tbsp of butter.
2. Once oil is hot, brown chicken for 5 minutes per side. Transfer to a plate and cut into strips.
3. In same pot, add remaining butter, sauté garlic for a minute until lightly browned.
4. Stir in paprika, cumin, coriander, turmeric, and garam masala. Sauté for a minute.
5. Stir in chicken and tomato paste. Sauté for 5 minutes. Season with salt.
6. Add water, bring to a simmer, cover, and cook for 10 minutes.
7. Add coconut milk and continue cooking for another 15 minutes.
8. Let it cool, evenly divide into suggested servings, and store in meal prep ready container.

Nutrition information:
Calories per serving: 520; Protein: 32.7g; Fat: 28g; Carbohydrates: 2.3g; Fiber: 0.8g

Chicken in Barbecue Chipotle Sauce

Serves: 6

Cooking Time: minutes

Ingredients:
- ¼ cup water
- ¼ teaspoon garlic powder
- ½ cup water
- 1 14-ounce boneless chicken breasts, skin removed
- 1 14-ounce boneless chicken thighs, skin removed
- 1 cup tomato sauce
- 1 onion, chopped
- 1/3 cup apple cider vinegar
- 2 tablespoons chipotle Tabasco sauce
- 2 tablespoons yellow mustard
- 4 tablespoons unsalted butter
- Salt and pepper to taste

Instructions:
1. In slow cooker, place all ingredients and mix well.
2. Cover and cook for 8 hours on low settings.
3. Let it cool, evenly divide into suggested servings, and store in meal prep ready container.

Nutrition information:
Calories per serving: 482; Protein: 29.4g; Fat: 18.7g; Carbohydrates: 3g; Fiber: 18.7g

Chicken Wings in 5-Spice Powder

Serves: 6

Cooking Time: 6 hours

Ingredients:

- ¼ teaspoon salt
- ¾ teaspoon red pepper flakes
- 1 tablespoon ginger, minced
- 1 tablespoon xanthan gum
- 1 teaspoon sesame oil
- 2 tablespoons Chinese five-spice powder
- 2 tablespoons garlic, minced
- 3 pounds chicken wings
- 3 tablespoons coconut aminos
- Toasted sesame seeds for garnish

Instructions:

1. Except for the sesame seeds, mix all ingredients thoroughly in the slow cooker.
2. Mix well. Cover and cook for 6 hours on low.
3. Let it cool, evenly divide into suggested servings, and store in meal prep ready container.

Nutrition information:

Calories per serving: 475; Protein: 31.8g; Fat: 21g; Carbohydrates: 3g; Fiber: 0.9g

Keto Meal-Prep Snacks Recipes

Dill & Tuna Topped Pickles

Serves: 5
Cooking Time: 0 minutes

Ingredients:
- Pepper and salt to taste
- 1 tbsp fresh dill, and more for garnish
- ¼ cup light mayo (sugar free)
- 1 can light flaked tuna, drained
- 5 dill pickles

Instructions:
1. Slice pickles in half, lengthwise. With a spoon, deseed the pickles and discard seeds.
2. In a small bowl, mix well the mayo, dill, and tuna using a fork.
3. Evenly divide the mixture into 10 and spread over deseeded pickles.
4. Garnish with more dill on top.
5. Evenly divide into suggested servings and store in meal prep ready container.

Nutrition information:
Calories per serving: 58; Protein: 7.6g; Fat: 1.1g; Carbohydrates: 5.8g; Fiber: 1.8g

Baked Parmesan Crisps

Serves: 10

Cooking Time: 10 minutes

Ingredients:

- 1 cup grated Parmesan cheese

Instructions:

6. Lightly grease a cookie sheet and preheat oven to 400°F.
7. Evenly sprinkle parmesan cheese on cookie sheet into 10 circles. Placing them about ½-inch apart.
8. Bake until lightly browned and crisped.
9. Let it cool, evenly divide into suggested servings, and store in meal prep ready container.

Nutrition information:

Calories per serving: 42; Protein: 2.8g; Fat: 2.8g; Carbohydrates: 1.4g; Fiber: 0g

Fudgy Snack Bombs

Serves: 30
Cooking Time: 5 minutes

Ingredients:
- 1 cup almond butter
- 1 cup coconut oil, at room temperature
- 1/16 tsp pink Himalayan salt
- 1/2 cup unsweetened cocoa powder
- 1/3 cup coconut flour
- 1/4 tsp powdered stevia

Instructions:
1. In a small pot on medium fire, melt and mix coconut oil and almond butter.
2. Once thoroughly combined, mix in the rest of the ingredients.
3. You can choose to roll the bombs in balls or pour them in a silicon mold.
4. If you want to pour it in molds, do it now and then freeze for 90 minutes.
5. If planning to roll, pour mixture in a bowl and let it freeze for 90 minutes. Afterwards, remove from freezer and roll into 30 balls.
6. Store in meal prep ready container.

Nutrition information:
Calories per serving: 117; Protein: 2.0g; Fat: 12.1g; Carbohydrates: 2.5g; Fiber: 1.3g

Pecan-Cinnamon Bars

Serves: 16
Cooking Time: 3 hours

Ingredients:

- ¼ cup heavy whipping cream
- ¼ teaspoon salt
- 1 ½ cups almond flour
- 1 cup pecans, chopped
- 1 cup stevia sweetener
- 1 tablespoon cinnamon
- 1 teaspoon baking powder
- 2 tablespoons unsalted butter
- 2 teaspoons vanilla extract
- 3 large eggs
- 6 tablespoons unsalted butter, melted

Instructions:

1. Grease the crockpot with butter.
2. In a bowl, combine the stevia sweetener and melted butter. Add in the eggs and vanilla extract.
3. Use a hand mixer to combine the ingredients.
4. In another bowl, combine the almond flour, salt, baking powder, and cinnamon.
5. Mix the wet ingredients to the dry ingredients until combined.
6. Pour the dough in the crockpot and press to form a dense bar.
7. Cook on low for 3 hours.
8. Meanwhile, mix the butter, whipping cream and pecans in a saucepan. Allow to boil and reduce slightly.
9. Once the bars are cooked, pour over the pecan sauce.
10. Let it cool, evenly divide into suggested servings, and store in meal prep ready container.

Nutrition information:

Calories per serving: 190.6; Protein: 4.4g; Fat: 20.6g; Carbohydrates: 1.9g; Fiber: 0g

Keto-Approved Brownies

Serves: 10
Cooking Time: 6 hours

Ingredients:

- ¾ cup coconut milk
- 2 tablespoons butter, melted
- 4 egg yolks, beaten
- 5 tablespoons cacao powder
- 1 teaspoon erythritol

Instructions:

1. In a bowl, mix well all ingredients.
2. Lightly grease your slow cooker with cooking spray and pour in batter.
3. Cover and cook on low for six hours.
4. Let it cool, evenly divide into suggested servings, and store in meal prep ready container.

Nutrition information:

Calories per serving: 84; Protein: 1.5g; Fat: 8.4g; Carbohydrates: 1.2g; Fiber: 0.8g

Chia Cinnamon Pudding

Serves: 2
Cooking Time: 0 minutes

Ingredients:
- 2 teaspoons unsweetened cacao powder
- 2 Tablespoons chia seeds
- Stevia to taste
- 1/2 teaspoon cinnamon powder
- 1/3 cup (78 ml) of coconut or almond milk
- 1/8 teaspoon vanilla extract

Instructions:
1. In a small bowl, mix well milk, vanilla, cinnamon, chia and cacao powder.
2. Refrigerate for 4 hours.
3. Evenly divide into suggested servings and store in meal prep ready container.

Nutrition information:
Calories per serving: 77; Protein: 3g; Fat: 5g; Carbohydrates: 6g; Fiber: 4g

Coconut Cream Cheese Cookies

Serves: 15
Cooking Time: 17 minutes

Ingredients:
- 1 Egg
- 1 teaspoon Vanilla extract
- 1/2 cup Butter softened
- 1/2 cup Coconut Flour
- 1/2 cup Erythritol or other sugar substitute
- 1/2 teaspoon baking powder
- 1/4 teaspoon salt
- 3 tablespoons Cream cheese, softened

Instructions:
1. In a mixing bowl, whisk well erythritol, cream cheese, and butter.
2. Add egg and vanilla. Beat until thoroughly combined.
3. Mix in salt, baking powder, and coconut flour.
4. On an 11x13-inch piece of wax paper, place the batter. Mold into a log shape and then twist the ends to secure. Refrigerate for an hour and then slice into 1-cm circles.
5. When ready, preheat oven to 350°F and line a baking sheet with foil. Place cookies at least 1/2-inch apart.
6. Pop in the oven and bake until golden brown, around 17 minutes.
7. Let it cool, evenly divide into suggested servings, and store in meal prep ready container.

Nutrition information:
Calories per serving: 91; Protein: 1g; Fat: 8g; Carbohydrates: 3g; Fiber: 2g

Rolled Deli Meat and Cheese

Serves: 6

Cooking Time: 0 minutes

Ingredients:
- 6 slices of all-natural turkey breast
- 3 slices of all-natural Colby jack cheese

Instructions:
1. Slice the cheese in half to make six slices.
2. On a flat surface, place 1 slice of turkey breast deli and add a slice of cheese.
3. Roll it up.
4. Repeat the process for remaining meat and cheese.
5. Store each roll in a meal prep ready container.

Nutrition information:
Calories per serving: 55; Protein: 5.0g; Fat: 3.6g; Carbohydrates: 0.5g; Fiber: 0g

Traditional Deviled Eggs

Serves: 12

Cooking Time: 10 minutes

Ingredients:

- 12 large eggs
- ¾ cup mayonnaise
- 1 tablespoon Dijon mustard
- Salt and pepper to taste
- Smoked paprika to taste
- 2 tablespoons pickle relish

Instructions:

1. In a large pot with 2-inches of water, add eggs and bring to a boil. Once boiling lower fire to medium and cook eggs for 8 minutes.
2. Drain water and run eggs under cold tap. Peel and slice lengthwise in half. Scoop out the yolk and place in a medium bowl.
3. In bowl of yolks, add remaining ingredients except for paprika and mix well. Evenly divide and place back in middle of egg whites. Sprinkle paprika on top.
4. Store in meal prep ready container.

Nutrition information:

Calories per serving: 132; Protein: 7.3g; Fat: 10.2g; Carbohydrates: 2.4g; Fiber: 0.4g

Mushrooms Stuffed with Pesto

Serves: 6
Cooking Time: 25 minutes

Ingredients:
- 6 large cremini mushrooms
- 6 bacon slices
- 2 tablespoons basil pesto
- 5 tablespoons cream cheese softened

Instructions:
1. Line a cookie sheet with foil and preheat oven to 375°F.
2. In a small bowl mix well, pesto and cream cheese.
3. Remove stems of mushrooms and discard. Evenly fill mushroom caps with pesto-cream cheese filling.
4. Get one stuffed mushroom and a slice of bacon. Wrap the bacon all over the mushrooms. Repeat process on remaining mushrooms and bacon.
5. Place bacon wrapped mushrooms on prepared pan and bake for 25 minutes or until bacon is crispy.
6. Let it cool, evenly divide into suggested servings, and store in meal prep ready container.

Nutrition information:
Calories per serving: 148; Protein: 4.9g; Fat: 13.9g; Carbohydrates: 1.4g; Fiber: 0.2g

Keto Meal-Prep Vegetarian/Vegetables Recipes

Roasted Herbed Veggies

Serves: 2

Cooking Time: 7 minutes

Ingredients:
- ¼ cup pepita seeds
- ¼ teaspoon salt
- ½ cup cherry tomatoes
- 1 green bell pepper, chopped
- 1 red bell pepper, chopped
- 1 teaspoon cumin
- 1 teaspoon dried oregano
- 1 yellow bell pepper, chopped
- 4 tablespoon olive oil
- 6 cups kale leaves, chopped

Instructions:
1. Lightly grease a cookie sheet and preheat oven to broil on low.
2. In a large bowl, mix well salt, cumin, oregano, and olive oil.
3. Add remaining ingredients and toss well to coat.
4. Place on prepared sheet and broil for 4 minutes. Remove from oven, toss or turnover and return to oven for another 3 minutes.
5. Let it cool, evenly divide into suggested servings, and store in meal prep ready container.

Nutrition information:
Calories per serving: 380; Protein: 8.6g; Fat: 35.8g; Carbohydrates: 13.8g; Fiber: 6.6g

Mac-Cauliflower and Cheese

Serves: 6

Cooking Time: 20 minutes

Ingredients:

- ½ cup nutritional yeast
- 1 ½ cup organic sharp cheddar cheese
- 1 ½ teaspoons Dijon mustard
- 1 cup heavy cream
- 1 large cauliflower, cut into 1/4-inch small florets
- 1 tablespoon garlic powder
- 2 ounces grass-fed cream cheese
- 2 tablespoons butter
- Salt and pepper to taste

Instructions:

1. Lightly grease an 11x13-inch rectangular baking dish and preheat oven to 350°F.
2. Evenly spread cauliflower in prepared dish. Season with pepper and salt.
3. In a medium microwave safe bowl, add butter and cream cheese. Microwave for 30 seconds and mix well. Stir in cheese, mustard, heavy cream, and garlic powder. Mix thoroughly. If needed, stick in microwave for a few seconds for easy handling and mixing.
4. Mix in yeast and pour over cauliflower. Toss well to coat.
5. Pop in the oven and bake until cauliflower is soft, around 15 to 20 minutes.
6. Let it cool, evenly divide into suggested servings, and store in meal prep ready container.

Nutrition information:

Calories per serving: 329; Protein: 16.1g; Fat: 25.5g; Carbohydrates: 10.8g; Fiber: 5.8g

Eggplant Salad Mediterranean Style

Serves: 2

Cooking Time: 15 minutes

Ingredients:

- 1 cup tomatoes, crushed
- 1 eggplant, quartered
- 1 red onion, sliced
- 1 tablespoon smoked paprika
- 2 bell peppers, sliced
- 2 teaspoons cumin
- 3 extra virgin olive oil
- Juice from 1 lemon, freshly squeezed
- Salt and pepper to taste

Instructions:

1. On medium high fire, place a medium pot. Heat oil.
2. Add tomatoes, eggplant, onion, bell peppers, and cumin. Stir fry for 5 minutes.
3. Add pepper and salt to taste.
4. Lower fire to medium, cover and cook for another 10 minutes.
5. Let it cool, evenly divide into suggested servings, and store in meal prep ready container.

Nutrition information:

Calories per serving: 312; Protein: 5.6g; Fat: 22g; Carbohydrates: 30.2g; Fiber: 27.1g

Stir-Fried Cabbage Asian Style

Serves: 4

Cooking Time: 7 minutes

Ingredients:

- ¼ teaspoon ground black pepper
- 1 2/3-pounds green cabbage
- 1 tablespoon fresh ginger, chopped into 3 pieces
- 1 tablespoon sesame oil
- 1 tablespoon white wine vinegar
- 1 teaspoon chili flakes
- 1 teaspoon onion powder
- 1 teaspoon salt
- 1/3-pound butter
- 2 garlic cloves, peeled, smashed and chopped
- 3 scallions

Instructions:

1. In food processor, shred cabbage until fine.
2. On medium high fire, place a large pan and heat ¼ of the butter.
3. Once butter is melted, stir fry cabbage for 5 minutes or until lightly browned but not soft.
4. Mix in white vinegar, black pepper, onion powder, and salt. Sauté for two minutes and transfer to a bowl.
5. Heat remaining butter and sauté fresh ginger, chili flakes, and garlic cloves.
6. Add cabbage back into pot.
7. Stir in scallions and mix well.
8. Taste and adjust seasoning if needed.
9. Drizzle with sesame oil, mix, and remove from pot.
10. Let it cool, evenly divide into suggested servings, and store in meal prep ready container.

Nutrition information:

Calories per serving: 370; Protein: 3.6g; Fat: 34.2g; Carbohydrates: 16.7g; Fiber: 4.7g

Vegetarian Casserole

Serves: 6

Cooking Time: minutes

Ingredients:

- ½ leek
- 1 cup heavy whipping cream
- 1-oz parmesan cheese, shredded
- 1 teaspoon onion powder
- ⅓ cup green olives
- 12 eggs
- 3-oz cherry tomatoes
- 7-oz shredded cheese
- salt and pepper

Instructions:

1. Lightly grease a 9x9-inch square baking dish and preheat oven to 400°F.
2. In a medium bowl, whisk eggs. Stir in onion powder and cream. Mix well.
3. Add the 7-oz shredded cheese in to the bowl and mix. Season with pepper and salt.
4. Evenly spread leeks and olives on prepared dish. Pour egg mixture over it.
5. Add the tomatoes.
6. Sprinkle parmesan on top and bake in the oven until tops are golden brown, around 35 minutes.
7. Let it cool, evenly divide into suggested servings, and store in meal prep ready container.

Nutrition information:

Calories per serving: 414; Protein: 22g; Fat: 34.7g; Carbohydrates: 4g; Fiber: 0.7g

Not So Ordinary Brussels Sprouts

Serves: 4
Cooking Time: 2 minutes

Ingredients:
- 1-pound Brussels sprouts, trimmed and cleaned
- ¼ cup pine nuts, toasted
- 1 pomegranate, seeds saved
- 1 tablespoon olive oil
- Salt and pepper
- 1 8-oz package sliced mushrooms
- 1 onion, sliced

Instructions:
1. Place a medium pan on medium-high fire and heat oil.
2. Once hot, stir fry onions for 3 minutes.
3. Add Brussels sprouts and mushrooms. Sauté for 10 minutes or until veggies are tender.
4. Stir in pine nuts and pomegranate seeds.
5. Season with pepper and salt to taste.
6. Let it cool, evenly divide into suggested servings, and store in meal prep ready container.

Nutrition information:
Calories per serving: 207; Protein: 7.9g; Fat: 10.5g; Carbohydrates: 26.5g; Fiber: 8g

Keto-Approved Stuffed Peppers

Serves: 4
Cooking Time: 40 minutes

Ingredients:
- ¼ cup baby spinach leaves
- ¼ teaspoon dried parsley
- ½ cup grated Parmesan cheese
- ½ cup ricotta cheese
- ½ cup shredded mozzarella
- 1 teaspoon garlic powder
- 2 medium bell peppers, sliced lengthwise in half and seeds removed
- 2 tablespoons Parmesan cheese, to garnish
- 4 large eggs

Instructions:
1. Lightly grease a cookie sheet with cooking spray and preheat oven to 375°F.
2. In a blender or food processor, mix parsley, garlic powder, eggs, and the three cheeses.
3. Evenly divide the cheese mixture and place them in the bell pepper cavities.
4. Add a couple spinach leaves on each pepper and mix them in with a fork.
5. Pop in the oven and bake until eggs have set, around 35 minutes.
6. Remove from oven and sprinkle parmesan on top. Return to oven and broil on high for 2 to 3 minutes.
7. Let it cool, evenly divide into suggested servings, and store in meal prep ready container.

Nutrition information:
Calories per serving: 245.5; Protein: 17.8g; Fat: 16.3g; Carbohydrates: 7.1g; Fiber: 1.1g

Cheese and Broccoli Fritters

Serves: 8

Cooking Time: 20 minutes

Ingredients:
- ¾ cup almond flour
- 2 large eggs
- 2 teaspoons baking powder
- 4 ounces fresh broccoli
- 4 ounces mozzarella cheese
- 7 tablespoons flaxseed meal
- Salt and Pepper to taste

Sauce Ingredients:
- ¼ cup fresh chopped dill
- ¼ cup mayonnaise
- ½ tablespoon lemon juice
- Salt and pepper to taste

Instructions:
1. In a food processor or blender, pulse broccoli until it is as fine as rice grains. Then, transfer to a large mixing bowl.
2. Stir in ¼ cup flaxseed meal, almond flour, and cheese. Season with pepper and salt.
3. Stir in eggs and mix well.
4. Evenly divide batter into 16 pieces and roll into balls. Then roll the balls in 3 tablespoons flaxseed meal.
5. Place a small deep pot on medium high fire and fill halfway up with oil for deep frying. If needed, deep fry the fritters in batches. Wait for the oil to heat before adding the fritters, around 10 minutes of heating.

6. Deep fry fritters until it turns golden brown, around 10 minutes.
7. Meanwhile, in a small bowl whisk well dill mayonnaise, and lemon juice. Season with pepper and salt.
8. Let it cool, evenly divide into suggested servings, place sauce on the side, and store in meal prep ready container.

Nutrition information:

Calories per serving: 207.8; Protein: g; Fat: 16.7g; Carbohydrates: 7.6g; Fiber: 3.8g

Zoodle Bowl with Sesame-Soy Dressing

Serves: 3

Cooking Time: 8 minutes

Ingredients:

- 2 medium zucchinis, spiralized
- ½ cup sliced mushrooms
- 1 cup shredded broccoli slaw mix
- 1 teaspoon sesame oil

Dressing Ingredients:

- ¼ cup almond butter
- ¼ teaspoon garlic powder
- 1 teaspoon crushed red pepper flakes
- 1 teaspoon erythritol
- 2 tablespoon chopped almonds, garnish
- 2 tablespoons sesame oil
- 2 tablespoons soy sauce

Instructions:

1. After the zucchinis are spiralized, squeeze out excess moisture or pat dry with paper towels and set aside.
2. On a large pan on medium fire, heat a teaspoon of sesame oil. Once hot, stir fry mushrooms for 3 minutes. Add shredded broccoli slaw mix and sauté for a minute or two until softened.
3. Add zoodles into pan and gently toss around with a fork until tender but not soggy, around 3 minutes.
4. Transfer to a bowl.
5. Meanwhile, mix well all dressing ingredients in a small bowl. Drizzle over zoodles and toss well to coat.
6. Let it cool, evenly divide into suggested servings, and store in meal prep ready container.

Nutrition information:

Calories per serving: 276; Protein: 8g; Fat: 24g; Carbohydrates: 11.9g; Fiber: 4.8g

Fresh Veggie Pizza

Serves: 2

Cooking Time: 20 minutes

Ingredients:
- ½ cup almond flour
- ½ teaspoon pepper
- ½ teaspoon salt
- 1 large egg
- 1 teaspoon Italian seasoning
- 2 tablespoons cream cheese
- 2 tablespoons fresh Parmesan cheese
- 2 tablespoons psyllium husk
- 6 ounces mozzarella cheese

Topping Ingredients:
- ¼ cup Rao's Marinara Sauce
- 1 medium vine tomato, sliced in circles
- 2/3 medium bell pepper, julienned
- 2-3 tablespoons fresh chopped basil
- 4 ounces shredded cheddar cheese

Instructions:
1. Preheat oven to 400°F.
2. In a mixing bowl, whisk well flour, pepper, salt, Italian seasoning, parmesan cheese, and psyllium husk. Add egg and mix a bit.
3. In a microwave safe bowl, add mozzarella and heat for 40 seconds or until pliable and melted. Stir in cream cheese and mix. Transfer to mixing bowl and mix in with your hands.

4. Evenly divide dough into two portions. Roll into a pizza crust to ¼-inch thick.

5. Once done rolling, bake in the oven until slightly golden brown, around ten minutes. Remove from oven and let it cool a bit.

6. Spread Marinara sauce on top of each crust. Evenly spread cheese. Add tomatoes, bell pepper, and basil.

7. Return to oven and bake until cheese has melted, around 8 minutes. And then turn broiler on and broil tops for 2 minutes or until bell pepper are a bit burned.

8. Let it cool, evenly divide into suggested servings, and store in meal prep ready container.

Nutrition information:

Calories per serving: 411.5; Protein: 22.3g; Fat: 31.3g; Carbohydrates: 12.5g; Fiber: 6.0g

Polenta with Sun-Dried Tomato

Serves: 4

Cooking Time: 25 minutes

Ingredients:

- ½ cup onion, chopped
- 1 bay leaf
- 1 cup polenta
- 1 teaspoon rosemary, chopped
- 1 teaspoon salt
- 1/3 cup sun-dried tomatoes, finely chopped
- 2 cloves of garlic, minced
- 2 tablespoons olive oil
- 2 tablespoons parsley, chopped
- 2 teaspoons oregano, chopped
- 3 tablespoons basil, chopped
- 4 cups vegetable stock

Instructions:

1. On a large pan on medium high fire, heat oil.
2. Sauté the garlic and onions for 3 minutes until fragrant.
3. Add sun-dried tomatoes, bay leaf, salt, parsley, oregano, basil, and rosemary. Stir to combine. And Sauté for 3 minutes.
4. Pour in stock and mix well.
5. Sprinkle polenta on top but do not stir.
6. Bring to a simmer, lower fire to medium, cover and cook for 15 minutes.
7. Let it cool, evenly divide into suggested servings, and store in meal prep ready container.

Nutrition information:

Calories per serving: 138; Protein: 2.1g; Fat: 7.2g; Carbohydrates: 17.0g; Fiber: 1.8g

Filling Mashed Sweet Potatoes

Serves: 8

Cooking Time: 40 minutes

Ingredients:
- ¼ cup milk
- ¼ teaspoon dried rosemary
- ¼ teaspoon dried sage
- ¼ teaspoon dried thyme
- ½ cup parmesan, grated
- ½ teaspoon dried parsley
- 1-pound sweet potatoes, peeled and cut into cubes
- 2 cloves of garlic
- 2 tablespoons butter
- Salt and pepper to taste

Instructions:
1. Fill a pot halfway up with water. Add well-scrubbed sweet potatoes and boil until soft, around 30 minutes.
2. To check if potatoes are tender, pierce with a fork and if it goes through easily it is ready. If not, continue boiling for another 10 minutes.
3. Drain potatoes and peel. Transfer to a bowl, mash and add remaining ingredients in bowl.
4. Mix well.
5. Let it cool, evenly divide into suggested servings, and store in meal prep ready container.

Nutrition information:
Calories per serving: 354; Protein: 4.1g; Fat: 21.7g; Carbohydrates: 35.4g; Fiber: 5.1g

Easy Steamed Vegetables

Serves: 4
Cooking Time: 10 minutes

Ingredients:
- ¼ cup parmesan cheese, grated
- ½ cup peeled garlic cloves
- 1 teaspoon Italian seasoning
- 2 bell peppers, sliced
- 2 large zucchinis, sliced
- 2 tablespoon olive oil
- Salt and pepper to taste

Instructions:
1. In a bowl, place peppers and zucchinis. Season with pepper, salt, Italian seasoning, garlic, and olive oil. Toss well to coat.
2. Transfer veggies on a steamer rack and sprinkle cheese on top.
3. Steam for 10 minutes.
4. Let it cool, evenly divide into suggested servings, and store in meal prep ready container.

Nutrition information:
Calories per serving: 190.5; Protein: 3g; Fat: 23.0g; Carbohydrates: 12.6g; Fiber: 9.1g

Stir Fried Summer Vegetables

Serves: 6

Cooking Time: 15 minutes

Ingredients:

- ½ cups balsamic vinegar
- ¼ cup olive oil
- 1 ½ cups onion, sliced
- 1 cup grape tomatoes
- 1 cup mushroom, sliced
- 1 tablespoon thyme, chopped
- 2 ½ cups zucchini, sliced
- 2 cups bell pepper, sliced
- 2 cups okra, sliced
- 2 tablespoons basil, chopped
- Salt and pepper

Instructions:

1. On medium high fire, place a medium pot and heat oil.
2. Once hot, stir in onions, mushrooms, thyme. Sauté for 5 minutes.
3. Season with pepper and salt.
4. Stir in bell pepper and okra. Sauté for 3 minutes.
5. Add balsamic vinegar, tomatoes, and zucchini. Cook for another 5 minutes.
6. Let it cool, evenly divide into suggested servings, and store in meal prep ready container.

Nutrition information:

Calories per serving: 233; Protein: 3g; Fat: 18g; Carbohydrates: 7g; Fiber: 4g

Zucchini Casserole

Serves: 4
Cooking Time: 35 minutes

Ingredients:
- 2 zucchinis, sliced
- 1 large onions, chopped
- 4 stalks celery, chopped
- 1 package of your favorite seasoning
- ½ cup vegetable stock
- 4 eggs, beaten
- Salt and pepper

Instructions:
1. Preheat oven to 350oF and lightly grease a medium casserole dish.
2. Evenly spread zucchinis, onions, and celery on bottom of casserole dish.
3. In a bowl beat eggs. Season with pepper and salt, generously.
4. In a cup mix vegetable stock and seasoning packet. Pour into egg mixture and beat well until thoroughly combined. Pour over vegetables in casserole dish and toss well to coat and mix.
5. Pop in the oven and bake until eggs are set, around 30 minutes.
6. If desired, you can turn on broiler and broil tops until golden brown around 2 to 3 minutes.
7. Let it cool, evenly divide into suggested servings, and store in meal prep ready container.

Nutrition information:
Calories per serving: 256; Protein: 5.7g; Fat: 2.4g; Carbohydrates: 14.2g; Fiber: 1.8g

Keto Meal-Prep Dessert Recipes

Mocha Flavored Pudding Cake

Serves: 9

Cooking Time: 20 minutes

Ingredients:

- ½ cup heavy cream
- ¾ cup butter
- 1 teaspoon vanilla extract
- 1/3 cup almond flour
- 1/8 teaspoon salt
- 2 tablespoons instant coffee crystals
- 2/3 cup granulated sweetener
- 2-ounces unsweetened chocolate
- 4 tablespoons unsweetened cocoa powder
- 5 large eggs
- Coconut oil spray

Instructions:

1. Lightly grease a 9x9-inch square pan and preheat oven to 350°F.
2. Place butter in a microwave safe bowl and melt. Once melted, stir in chocolate and mix well. If needed, heat again in 10-second intervals to melt the chocolate.
3. In a mixing bowl, whisk well the eggs until pale. Slowly add the sweetener while beating continuously.
4. Beat in heavy cream, coffee crystals, and vanilla.
5. Beat in melted butter and chocolate mixture.
6. Stir in cocoa powder, almond flour, and salt. Mix thoroughly.
7. Pour batter into prepared pan and bake in the oven for 20 minutes.
8. Let it cool, evenly divide into suggested servings, and store in meal prep ready container.

Nutrition information:

Calories per serving: 265.7; Protein: 2.4g; Fat: 20.8g; Carbohydrates: 18.6g; Fiber: 0.9g

Keto-Approved Lemon Bars

Serves: 12
Cooking Time: 25 minutes

Ingredients:
- ¼ cup cashew
- ¼ cup fresh lemon juice, freshly squeezed
- ¾ cup coconut milk
- ¾ cup erythritol
- 1 cup desiccated coconut
- 1 teaspoon baking powder
- 2 eggs, beaten
- 2 tablespoons coconut oil
- A dash of salt

Instructions:
1. Preheat oven to 350°F and lightly grease an 8x8-inch square pan.
2. Combine thoroughly all ingredients in a mixing bowl.
3. Pour batter in prepared pan and bake for 20-25 minutes.
4. Let it cool, evenly divide into suggested servings, and store in meal prep ready container.

Nutrition information:
Calories per serving: 113; Protein: 2.6g; Fat: 10.2g; Carbohydrates: 3.9g; Fiber: 1.7g

Doubly Dark Choco Cake

Serves: 8

Cooking Time: 30 minutes

Ingredients:

- ¼ cups unsweetened applesauce
- ½ cup cacao powder
- ½ cup coconut milk, full fat
- ½ teaspoon vanilla
- 1 cup almond flour
- 1 large egg
- 2 tablespoons almond milk, unsweetened
- 2 tablespoons raw cacao nibs
- 2 tablespoons tapioca flour
- 2 tablespoons stevia

Instructions:

1. Preheat oven to 350°F and lightly grease an 8-inch round pan.
2. In a large mixing bowl, whisk well egg. Sit in applesauce, coconut milk, vanilla, almond milk, and stevia. Mix well.
3. Stir in cocoa powder, almond flour, and tapioca flour. And mix well.
4. Pour into prepared pan and bake until set, around 30 minutes.
5. To test for doneness, stick a toothpick in middle of cake and if it comes out clean then the cake is cooked.
6. Remove from oven.
7. Let it cool, evenly divide into suggested servings, and store in meal prep ready container.

Nutrition information:

Calories per serving: 90; Protein: 2.1g; Fat: 6.6g; Carbohydrates: 16.0g; Fiber: 2.4g

Easy Cheesecake in Pressure Cooker

Serves: 16

Cooking Time: 30 minutes

Ingredients:

- 3 8-ounce cream cheese, room temperature
- 1 cup stevia
- 3 eggs
- ½ tablespoon vanilla extract

Instructions:

1. Line a spring form pan with foil. Make sure that the pan can fit inside your pressure cooker.
2. In a blender, mix all ingredients until smooth and creamy.
3. Pour into prepared pan. Cover top securely with foil.
4. In pressure cooker, add a cup or two of water. Place a trivet and put the pan on the trivet.
5. Cover and pressure cook for 25 minutes and let pressure release naturally.
6. Let it cool, evenly divide into suggested servings, and store in meal prep ready container.

Nutrition information:

Calories per serving: 138.5; Protein: 4.0g; Fat: 13.0g; Carbohydrates: 3.4g; Fiber: 0g

Keto-Approved Pecan Blondie Bars

Serves: 16

Cooking Time: 30 minutes

Ingredients:

- ¼ cup heavy whipping cream
- ¼ teaspoon salt
- 1 ½ cups all-purpose flour
- 1 cup pecans, chopped
- ¾ cup stevia
- 1 tablespoon cinnamon
- 1 teaspoon baking powder
- 2 teaspoon vanilla extract
- 3 large eggs
- 6 tablespoons unsalted butter, melted

Instructions:

1. Preheat oven to 350°F and lightly grease a medium rectangular baking pan.
2. In a large mixing bowl, whisk well eggs until fluffy.
3. Stir in whipping cream, salt, stevia, baking powder, butter, and vanilla. Mix thoroughly.
4. Add remaining ingredients and mix thoroughly.
5. Pour in prepared pan and pop in the oven.
6. Bake for 30 minutes or until when toothpick is inserted in the middle comes out clean.
7. Let it cool, evenly divide into suggested servings, and store in meal prep ready container.

Nutrition information:

Calories per serving: 190.6; Protein: 4.4g; Fat: 20.6g; Carbohydrates: 1.9g; Fiber: 0g

Raspberry Coconut Slice

Serves: 20
Cooking Time: 30 minutes

Ingredients:

- 1 cup raspberries
- 1 teaspoon powdered erythritol
- 3 tablespoons chia seeds
- 2 tablespoons water
- 4 ounces 85% dark chocolate

Coconut Layer Ingredients:

- 1 cup coconut milk, unsweetened, canned
- ¼ cup coconut oil
- 3 cups desiccated coconut, unsweetened
- 1/3 cup powdered erythritol
- 1 teaspoon vanilla bean powder
- Pinch of sea salt

Biscuit Layer Ingredients:

- 2 cups almond meal
- ½ teaspoon baking soda
- 1 tablespoon butter, room temperature
- 1 large egg

Instructions:

1. Lightly grease an 8x8-inch baking pan and preheat oven to 350°F.
2. In a small bowl, mix the biscuit layer ingredients. Press on bottom of prepared pan and bake until lightly browned around 15 minutes. Remove from oven and cool.

3. On low heat, place a small pot and make the raspberry layer. Add raspberries, erythritol, chia seeds, and water. Break the raspberries to make a puree while cooking until thickened, around 5 minutes.

4. In another small pot, make the coconut layer by heating coconut milk and oil on medium fire for 5 minutes. Mix in desiccated coconut, erythritol, vanilla bean, and salt. Mix well and turn off fire. Pour over biscuit layer and place in the freezer to harden for at least an hour.

5. Once the coconut layer has hardened, spread the raspberry layer on top of it and freeze again for another hour.

6. Meanwhile, melt dark chocolate in microwave. Spread on top of raspberry layer and chill in the fridge for 30 minutes.

7. Evenly divide into suggested servings and store in meal prep ready container.

Nutrition information:

Calories per serving: 241.5; Protein: 4.6g; Fat: 22.2g; Carbohydrates: 8.8g; Fiber: 5.3g

Coconut-Lime Bars

Serves: 16
Cooking Time: 25 minutes

Ingredients:

- 4 eggs
- 1 tablespoon lime zest
- 1/2 cup lime juice
- 1/2 teaspoon coconut stevia
- 1/4 cup sesame flour or almond flour
- 1 1/4 cup Swerve sweetener divided
- 1/4 teaspoon sea salt
- 1/4 cup coconut oil room temperature
- 1/4 cup unsweetened coconut flakes
- 3/4 cup coconut flour

Instructions:

1. Lightly grease an 8x8-inch baking pan and preheat oven to 350°F.
2. In a blender, pulse coconut oil, salt, ¼ cup swerve sweetener, sesame flour, and coconut flour. Press on bottom of prepared pan. Bake until lightly browned, around 10 minutes.
3. Meanwhile, in a bowl, whisk well coconut stevia, 1 cup Swerve, lime zest, lime juice, add eggs. Pour this on baked crust.
4. Evenly spread coconut flakes on top and pop in the oven until the center is set, around 13 to 15 minutes.
5. Let it cool, evenly divide into suggested servings, and store in meal prep ready container.

Nutrition information:

Calories per serving: 100; Protein: 3.5g; Fat: 7.2g; Carbohydrates: 5.7g; Fiber: 2.5g

Choco-Coco Bars

Serves: 12

Cooking Time: 0 minutes

Ingredients:

- 3 squares Baker's Unsweetened Chocolate (3 ounces chocolate)
- 1 tablespoon coconut oil
- 2 droppers Liquid Stevia
- 2 cups shredded unsweetened coconut
- 1/3 c Virgin Coconut Oil, melted
- 2 droppers of Liquid Stevia (or enough sweetener to equal 1/4 cup)

Instructions:

1. Lightly grease an 8x8-inch silicone pan.
2. In a food processor, process shredded unsweetened coconut, coconut oil, and Stevia until it forms a dough. Transfer to prepared pan and press on bottom to form a dough. Place in the freezer to set.
3. Meanwhile, in a microwave safe Pyrex cup, place chocolate, coconut oil, and Stevia. Heat for 10-second intervals and mix well. Do not overheat, just until you have mixed the mixture thoroughly. Pour over dough.
4. Return to freezer until set.
5. Evenly divide into suggested servings, and store in meal prep ready container.

Nutrition information:

Calories per serving: 216; Protein: 2g; Fat: 22g; Carbohydrates: 4g; Fiber: 2g

Keto Carrot-Cake Balls

Serves: 16
Cooking Time: 0 minutes

Ingredients:
- 1 (8-oz) block cream cheese, softened
- 1 teaspoon stevia
- 1 teaspoon cinnamon
- 1 cup grated carrots
- 1 cup shredded unsweetened coconut
- 1/2 teaspoon pure vanilla extract
- 1/2 cup chopped pecans
- 1/4 teaspoon ground nutmeg
- 3/4 cup coconut flour

Instructions:
1. In a medium mixing bowl, beat cream cheese, stevia, cinnamon, vanilla, nutmeg, and coconut flour.
2. Fold in pecans and carrots.
3. Evenly divide into 16 portions and roll into balls. Roll balls until covered with shredded coconut.
4. Store in meal prep ready container.

Nutrition information:
Calories per serving: 101; Protein: 1.7g; Fat: 8.6g; Carbohydrates: 5.5g; Fiber: 1g

Fudgy Brownies with Avocado

Serves: 12

Cooking Time: 35 minutes

Ingredients:

- 250 g avocado about 2
- 4 tbsp cocoa powder
- 1 tsp stevia powder
- 3 tbsp refined coconut oil
- 2 eggs
- 100 g lily's dark chocolate melted
- 90 g blanched almond flour
- 1 tsp baking powder
- 1/2 tsp vanilla
- 1/4 tsp baking soda
- 1/4 tsp salt
- 1/4 cup erythritol

Instructions:

1. Lightly grease a 9x9-inch baking pan and preheat oven to 350°F.
2. In a blender or food processor, process the avocados until smooth.
3. Add eggs, coconut oil, salt, vanilla, baking soda, baking powder, erythritol, and melted chocolate. Process again until smooth.
4. Add cocoa powder and almond flour. Process until smooth.
5. Transfer to prepared pan.
6. Bake for 35 minutes.
7. Let it cool, evenly divide into suggested servings, and store in meal prep ready container.

Nutrition information:

Calories per serving: 158; Protein: 3.8g; Fat: 14.3g; Carbohydrates: 9.0g; Fiber: 6.6g

Ketogenic Diet 4-Week Meal Plan

Week 1: Shopping List

- 1 ½ lbs beef round steak
- 1 bottle almond butter
- 1 bottle apple cider vinegar
- 1 bottle coconut oil
- 1 bottle Dijon mustard
- 1 bottle dill pickles
- 1 bottle green pesto
- 1 bottle ketchup
- 1 bottle nutritional yeast
- 1 bottle prepared mustard
- 1 bottle sesame oil
- 1 bottle soy sauce
- 1 bottle vanilla extract
- 1 bottle vinegar
- 1 can flaked tuna
- 1 can pitted olive
- 1 eggplant, large
- 1 kg almond flour
- 1 large carrot
- 1 large ginger
- 1 lb red tomatoes
- 1 pack baking powder
- 1 pack cashew
- 1 pack cheddar cheese
- 1 pack coconut flour
- 1 pack dark chocolate
- 1 pack desiccated coconut
- 1 pack erythritol
- 1 pack Himalayan salt
- 1 pack instant coffee
- 1 pack mayonnaise
- 1 pack Mexican cheese
- 1 pack raw cacao nibs
- 1 pack sambal paste
- 1 pack stevia
- 1 pack tapioca flour
- 1 pack turkey ham
- 1 small carton of milk
- 1 small pack sour cream
- 1 yellow bell pepper
- 100 g pepita seeds
- 1kg Mozzarella cheese
- 2 blocks cream cheese
- 2 head broccolis
- 2 lbs beef brisket
- 2 pounds salmon fillet

- 2 red bell peppers
- 2 sirloin steaks
- 250 g Colby Jack cheese
- 250 g parmesan cheese, grated
- 3 bottles coconut cream
- 3 cans tomato sauce
- 3 green bell peppers
- 3 lbs ground beef
- 3 lemons
- 3.5 lbs butter
- 3lbs chicken breasts
- 4 cans heavy cream
- 4 pcs chicken legs
- 4 pork chops, boneless
- 5 heads of cabbage
- 500 g Feta cheese
- 500 mL almond milk
- 60 eggs
- 7 garlic bulbs
- 7 large onions
- 8 bacon slices
- 8 ounces mushrooms
- applesauce, sugar-free
- baby kale
- bay leaves

- black pepper
- cherry tomatoes
- chili flakes
- cranberry sauce, sugar-free
- cumin powder
- dried oregano
- dried rosemary
- dried tarragon
- dried thyme
- dried thyme
- five spice powder
- fresh basil
- fresh dill
- fresh parsley
- garam masala
- garlic powder
- green onions
- olive oil
- onion powder
- red pepper
- salt
- smoked paprika
- spinach leaves
- star anise
- whole pepper corn

Week 1: Meal Plan

Day 1

Breakfast: Beef and Egg White Scramble
Lunch: Slow Cooked Corned Beef
Dinner: Chicken Marsala Casserole
Snacks/Dessert: Mocha Flavored Pudding Cake

Day 2

Breakfast: Breakfast Muffin Cups
Lunch: Roasted Herbed Veggies
Dinner: Beef Brisket with Cranberry Gravy
Snacks/Dessert: Keto-Approved Lemon Bars

Day 3

Breakfast: Ketogenic Quiche
Lunch: Keto Swiss Steak
Dinner: Mac-Cauliflower and Cheese
Snacks/Dessert: Dill & Tuna Topped Pickles

Day 4

Breakfast: Ketogenic Fried Bacon and Eggs
Lunch: Traditional Filipino Adobo
Dinner: Baked Herbed Salmon
Snacks/Dessert: Baked Parmesan Crisps

Day 5

Breakfast: Spinach and Egg-white Omelet

Lunch: Ginger Beef Asian Style
Dinner: Eggplant Salad Mediterranean Style
Snacks/Dessert: Fudgy Snack Bombs

Day 6

Breakfast: Feta-Kale Egg Casserole
Lunch: Stir-Fried Cabbage Asian Style
Dinner: Asian-Inspired Keto Pork Chops
Snacks/Dessert: Doubly Dark Choco Cake

Day 7

Breakfast: Cream Cheese & Mushroom Egg Casserole
Lunch: Ground Beef and Cabbage Stir-Fry
Dinner: Pesto Chicken Casserole
Snacks/Dessert: Mocha Flavored Pudding Cake

Week 2: Shopping List

- ½ lb bacon
- ½ lb blue cheese
- ½ lb mushrooms
- ½ lb potatoes
- ½ lbs tomatoes
- ½ leek
- 1 bottle avocado oil
- 1 bottle capers
- 1 bottle green olives
- 1 bottle white wine
- 1 bottle Worcestershire sauce
- 1 carton of milk
- 1 chipotle pepper
- 1 head cauliflower
- 1 knob ginger, large
- 1 lb Brussels sprouts
- 1 lb cod fillet
- 1 pack arugula
- 1 pack cottage cheese
- 1 pack kale
- 1 pack psyllium husk powder
- 1 pomegranate
- 1 shallot
- 1 sprig fresh dill
- 1 whole chicken
- 100 g pepper jack cheese
- 100 g raspberries
- 100 g ricotta cheese
- 2 ½ lb chicken breasts
- 2 apricots
- 2 cans diced tomatoes
- 2 cans sour cream
- 2 lbs beef roast
- 2 lbs goat meat
- 2 lbs ground beef
- 2 lemons
- 250 g sun-dried tomatoes
- 3 cans coconut milk
- 3 garlic bulbs
- 4 6-oz salmon fillets
- 4 cans heavy cream
- 4 oz dark chocolate
- 4 sticks butter
- 4 zucchinis
- 5 onions
- 5 yellow onion
- 65 eggs
- 750 g grated parmesan
- 750 g pecans
- 8 green bell peppers
- 8 oz crab meat
- 8 oz cream cheese
- 8 oz sausage
- black olives

- cardamom pods
- chia
- chili powder
- cinnamon
- cloves
- coriander powder
- dried parsley

- flaxseed
- frozen spinach
- hot sauce
- lemongrass stalk
- pine nuts
- sunflower seeds
- turmeric

Week 2: Meal Plan

Day 1

Breakfast: Cauliflower Breakfast Quiche
Lunch: Goat Curry Mediterranean Style
Dinner: Vegetarian Casserole
Snacks/Dessert: Easy Cheesecake in Pressure Cooker

Day 2

Breakfast: Breakfast Burger in Slow Cooker
Lunch: Creamy Crab-Spinach Bake
Dinner: Slow-Cooked Beef Moroccan Style
Snacks/Dessert: Keto-Approved Pecan Blondie Bars

Day 3

Breakfast: Baked Eggs Greek Style
Lunch: Beef Stroganoff Keto Style
Dinner: Not So Ordinary Brussels Sprouts
Snacks/Dessert: Pecan-Cinnamon Bars

Day 4

Breakfast: Egg and Sausage Sandwich
Lunch: Keto-Approved Stuffed Peppers
Dinner: Baked Cod Topped with Arugula Tapenade
Snacks/Dessert: Keto-Approved Brownies

Day 5

Breakfast: Keto-Approved Breakfast Pizza
Lunch: Baked Salmon Topped with Caper-Relish
Dinner: Ground Beef and Cheese Casserole
Snacks/Dessert: Chia Cinnamon Pudding

Day 6

Breakfast: Keto-Approved Pancakes
Lunch: Stir-Fried Cabbage Asian Style
Dinner: Chicken in Coco-Turmeric Sauce
Snacks/Dessert: Raspberry Coconut Slice

Day 7

Breakfast: Keto-Approved Breakfast Porridge
Lunch: Fajita Chicken
Dinner: Zucchini and Cheese Gratin
Snacks/Dessert: Keto-Approved Pecan Blondie Bars

Week 3: Shopping List

- 1 ½ lb chicken breasts
- 1 beef shoulder
- 1 bottle coconut aminos
- 1 can coconut cream
- 1 celery stalk
- 1 cup broccoli slaw mix
- 1 jalapeno pepper
- 1 large tomato
- 1 pack almond nuts
- 1 pack cherry tomatoes
- 1 pack dried tomatoes
- 1 pack Italian seasoning
- 1 pack polenta
- 1 pack spinach
- 1 yellow squash
- 2 cans heavy cream
- 2 carrots
- 2 lbs ground beef
- 2 shallots
- 2 small heads broccoli
- 2 sprigs cilantro leaves
- 2 sprigs green onion
- 2 stalks lemon grass
- 20 oz cream cheese
- 250 g cheddar cheese
- 250 g Colby jack cheese
- 3 garlic bulbs
- 3 packs spinach
- 3 zucchinis
- 4 lbs baby back ribs
- 4 lbs pork shoulder
- 4 limes
- 4 pork loin chops
- 4 salmon fillets
- 5 lemons
- 5 onions
- 5 oz baby kale
- 5 oz Feta cheese
- 5 sticks of butter
- 6 dried birds eye chilies
- 6 kaffir lime leaves
- 6 slices turkey breasts
- 6 slices turkey ham
- 6 sweet peppers
- 62 eggs
- 8 beef steaks
- 8 oz mushrooms
- 8 slices of bacon
- A sprig of fresh basil
- cayenne powder
- nutmeg
- oyster sauce

Week 3: Meal Plan

Day 1

Breakfast: Bacon and Cheese Stuffed Peppers
Lunch: Vegetable-Chicken Creamy Casserole
Dinner: Porkchops with Rosemary-Garlic Blend
Snacks/Dessert: Coconut-Lime Bars

Day 2

Breakfast: Beef and Egg White Scramble
Lunch: Cheese and Broccoli Fritters
Dinner: Easy Meatballs
Snacks/Dessert: Choco-Coco Bars

Day 3

Breakfast: Breakfast Muffin Cups
Lunch: Slow Cooked Pork Carnitas
Dinner: Herbed-Crusted Baked Salmon
Snacks/Dessert: Coconut Cream Cheese Cookies

Day 4

Breakfast: Ketogenic Quiche
Lunch: Zoodle Bowl with Sesame-Soy Dressing
Dinner: Pork Ribs in Slow Cooker
Snacks/Dessert: Rolled Deli Meat and Cheese

Day 5

Breakfast: Ketogenic Fried Bacon and Eggs
Lunch: Malaysian Style Beef Stew
Dinner: Fresh Veggie Pizza
Snacks/Dessert: Traditional Deviled Eggs

Day 6

Breakfast: Spinach and Egg-white Omelet
Lunch: Creamy Chicken Tuscan Style
Dinner: Stir-Fried Mushrooms and Beef
Snacks/Dessert: Choco-Coco Bars

Day 7

Breakfast: Feta-Kale Egg Casserole
Lunch: Beef Steak Filipino Style
Dinner: Polenta with Sun-Dried Tomato
Snacks/Dessert: Keto Carrot-Cake Balls

Week 4: Shopping List

- ¼ cup coconut oil
- ½ lbs potatoes
- 1 bottle avocado oil
- 1 bottle balsamic vinegar
- 1 bottle Tabasco sauce
- 1 can tomato sauce
- 1 can whipping cream
- 1 carton milk
- 1 head cauliflower
- 1 head of cabbage
- 1 large knob of ginger
- 1 lb sweet potatoes
- 1 pack all spice
- 1 pack dried sage
- 1 pack tomato paste
- 1 pack xanthan gum
- 100 g Mexican cheese blend
- 12 oz cream cheese
- 14 oz cherry tomatoes
- 14 oz okra
- 2 cans coconut milk
- 2 cans heavy cream
- 2 lbs goat meat
- 2 slices cheddar cheese
- 2.5 lbs chicken breasts
- 2.5 lbs chicken thighs
- 20 oz sausages
- 3 lbs chicken wings
- 3 lbs ground beef
- 3 sprigs scallions
- 4 garlic bulbs
- 4 large zucchinis
- 4 oz fresh blueberries
- 4 oz sun-dried tomatoes
- 4 sticks butter
- 5 onions
- 6 bacon slices
- 6 large cremini mushrooms
- 7 bell peppers
- 78 eggs
- 8 oz Feta cheese
- 8 oz mushrooms
- 8 oz pepper jack cheese
- 8 oz raspberries
- A sprig of fresh basil
- A sprig of fresh thyme
- toasted sesame seeds

Week 4: Meal Plan

Day 1

Breakfast: Cream Cheese & Mushroom Egg Casserole
Lunch: Tender Jerk Chicken
Dinner: Filling Mashed Sweet Potatoes
Snacks/Dessert: Keto-Approved Pecan Blondie Bars

Day 2

Breakfast: Cauliflower Breakfast Quiche
Lunch: Chicken Marsala Casserole
Dinner: Buttered Chicken from India
Snacks/Dessert: Raspberry Coconut Slice

Day 3

Breakfast: Breakfast Burger in Slow Cooker
Lunch: Chicken in Barbecue Chipotle Sauce
Dinner: Easy Steamed Vegetables
Snacks/Dessert: Mushrooms Stuffed with Pesto

Day 4

Breakfast: Baked Eggs Greek Style
Lunch: Stir Fried Summer Vegetables
Dinner: Chicken Wings in 5-Spice Powder
Snacks/Dessert: Mocha Flavored Pudding Cake

Day 5

Breakfast: Egg and Sausage Sandwich
Lunch: Slow Cooked Corned Beef
Dinner: Traditional Filipino Adobo
Snacks/Dessert: Coconut-Lime Bars

Day 6

Breakfast: Keto-Approved Breakfast Pizza
Lunch: Zucchini Casserole
Dinner: Ginger Beef Asian Style
Snacks/Dessert: Choco-Coco Bars

Day 7

Breakfast: Keto-Approved Pancakes
Lunch: Ground Beef and Cabbage Stir-Fry
Dinner: Goat Curry Mediterranean Style
Snacks/Dessert: Mushrooms Stuffed with Pesto

Conclusion

A ketogenic diet comes with a lot of benefits. It is a practical approach to weight loss. Meal prepping ensures your success while following the ketogenic diet. Although it needs a lot of careful planning and execution, you can still save time and effort compared to making meals every day. After reading this eBook, if you are overwhelmed with the information it contains rest assured that these tips are here to help you navigate your way through this wonderful and effective diet regimen.

The purpose of meal prepping is not only for convenience, but it can help ensure that you are following the principles of the ketogenic diet. After all, achieving the state of ketosis is difficult, especially if you are not minding your macros. Thus, meal prepping is also all about enforcing self-discipline to not consume foods that you did not prepare. It basically keeps you on the right track so that you can achieve your weight loss goals.

Let me remind you though that unlike other fad diets, it might take several weeks or months for you to see drastic results so do not falter. Keep going. Know that you are not alone in this journey.

Made in the USA
Lexington, KY
11 March 2019